Underground Clinical Vignettes

Pathophysiology III: CV, Dermatology, GU, Orthopedic, General Surgery, Peds

FIFTH EDITION

Underground Clinical Vignettes

Pathophysiology III: CV, Dermatology, GU, Orthopedic, General Surgery, Peds

FIFTH EDITION

Todd A. Swanson, M.D., Ph.D.
Resident in Radiation Oncology
William Beaumont Hospital
Royal Oak, Michigan

Sandra I. Kim, M.D., Ph.D.
Resident in Internal Medicine
Beth Israel Deaconess Medical Center
Harvard Medical School
Boston, Massachusetts

Olga E. Flomin, M.D.
Resident in Obstetrics and Gynecology
William Beaumont Hospital
Royal Oak, Michigan

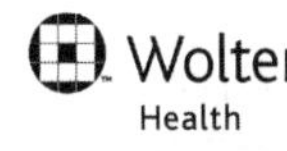

Wolters Kluwer | Lippincott Williams & Wilkins
Health
Philadelphia • Baltimore • New York • London
Buenos Aires • Hong Kong • Sydney • Tokyo

Acquisitions Editor: Nancy Anastasi Duffy
Developmental Editor: Kathleen H. Scogna
Managing Editor: Nancy Hoffmann
Marketing manager: Jennifer Kuklinski
Assistant Production Manager: Kevin Johnson
Creative Director: Doug Smock
Compositor: International Typesetting and Composition
Printer: R.R. Donnelley & Son's: Crawfordsville

351 West Camden Street
Baltimore, MD 21201

530 Walnut Street
Philadelphia, PA 19106

Printed in the United States of America

First Edition, 2001 Blackwell Publishing Inc.
Second Edition, 2003 Blackwell Publishing Inc.
Third Edition, 2005 Blackwell Publishing Inc.
Fourth Edition, 2005 Blackwell Publishing Inc.

Library of Congress Cataloging-in-Publication Data

Swanson, Todd A.
Pathophysiology. III, CV, dermatology, GU, orthopedic, general surgery, peds / Todd Swanson, Sandra Kim, Olga E. Flomin.—5th ed.
p. ; cm.—(Underground clinical vignettes)
Rev. ed. of: Pathophysiology / Tao Le . . . [et al.]. 4th ed. c2005.
Includes bibliographical references and index.
ISBN-13: 978-0-7817-6468-1
ISBN-10: 0-7817-6468-8
1. Physiology, Pathological—Case studies. 2. Physicians—Licenses—United States—Examinations—Study guides. I. Kim, Sandra. II. Flomin, Olga E. III. Pathophysiology. IV. Title. V. Title: CV, dermatology, GU, orthopedic, general surgery, peds. VI. Series.
[DNLM: 1. Clinical Medicine—Case Reports. 2. Clinical Medicine—Problems and Exercises. WB 18.2 S9725pb 2007]
RB113.B459 2007
616.07076—dc22

2007001466

To purchase additional copies of this book, call our customer service department at **(800) 638-3030** or fax orders to **(301) 223-2320.** International customers should call **(301) 223-2300.**

Visit Lippincott Williams & Wilkins on the Internet: http://www.LWW.com. Lippincott Williams & Wilkins customer service representatives are available from 8:30 am to 6:00 pm, EST.

07 08 09 10
1 2 3 4 5 6 7 8 9 10

dedication

For T.M.

preface

First published in 1999, the Underground Clinical Vignettes series has provided thousands of students with a highly effective review tool as they prepare for medical exams, particularly the USMLE Step 1 and 2 exams. Designed as a quick study guide, each UCV book contains patient-centered clinical cases that highlight a range of medical diagnoses.

With this new edition of Underground Clinical Vignettes, we have incorporated feedback from medical students across the country to provide updated cases with expanded treatment and discussion sections. A new two-page format enables readers to formulate an initial diagnosis prior to reading the answer, while the added differential diagnosis section encourages critical thinking about comparable cases. The inclusion of relevant MRI images, radiographs, and photographs allows students to visualize the physical presentation of each case more readily. Breakout points, tables, and algorithms have been added, along with all new Board-format QAs, making this edition of UCV an ideal source of information for exam review, classroom discussion, or clinical rotations.

The clinical vignettes in this series are designed to give added emphasis to pathogenesis, epidemiology, management, and complications. Although each case tends to present all the signs, symptoms, and diagnostic findings for a particular illness, patients generally will not present with such a "complete" picture either clinically or on a medical examination. Cases are not meant to simulate a potential real patient or an exam vignette.

Access to the LWW online companion site, ThePoint, will be offered as a premium with the purchase of the Underground Clinical Vignettes Step 1 bundle. Benefits include an online test link and additional new Board-format questions covering all UCV subject areas.

We hope you will find the Underground Clinical Vignettes series informative and useful. We welcome any feedback, suggestions, or corrections you have about this series. Please contact us at LWW.com/medstudent.

contributors

Series Editors

Todd A. Swanson, M.D., Ph.D.
Resident in Radiation Oncology
William Beaumont Hospital
Royal Oak, Michigan

Sandra I. Kim, M.D., Ph.D.
Resident in Internal Medicine
Beth Israel Deaconess Medical Center
Harvard Medical School
Boston, Massachusetts

Series Contributors

Olga E. Flomin, M.D.
Resident in Obstetrics and Gynecology
William Beaumont Hospital
Royal Oak, Michigan

Medina C. Kushen, M.D.
Resident in Neurosurgery
University of Chicago Hospitals
Chicago, Illinois

Marc J. Glucksman, Ph.D.
Professor of Biochemistry and Molecular Biology
Director, Midwest Proteome Center and
Co-Director, Rosalind Franklin Structural Biology Laboratories
Rosalind Franklin University of Medicine and Science
The Chicago Medical School
North Chicago, Illinois

acknowledgments

Thanks to Dr. Alvaro Martinez, Dr. Larry Kestin and the entire radiation oncology program at William Beaumont Hospital for allowing the flexibility to work on this project during an already vigorous residency training program.

—Todd A. Swanson

Thanks to Todd for his work on this series.

—Sandra I. Kim

abbreviations

ABGs	arterial blood gases
ABPA	allergic bronchopulmonary aspergillosis
ACA	anticardiolipin antibody
ACE	angiotensin-converting enzyme
ACL	anterior cruciate ligament
ACTH	adrenocorticotropic hormone
AD	adjustment disorder
ADA	adenosine deaminase
ADD	attention-deficit disorder
ADH	antidiuretic hormone
ADHD	attention-deficit–hyperactivity disorder
ADP	adenosine diphosphate
AFO	ankle-foot orthosis
AFP	α-fetoprotein
AIDS	acquired immunodeficiency syndrome
ALL	acute lymphocytic leukemia
ALS	amyotrophic lateral sclerosis
ALT	alanine aminotransferase
AML	acute myelogenous leukemia
ANA	antinuclear antibody
Angio	angiography
AP	anteroposterior
APKD	adult polycystic kidney disease
aPTT	activated partial thromboplastin time
ARDS	adult respiratory distress syndrome
5-ASA	5-aminosalicylic acid
ASCA	antibodies to *Saccharomyces cerevisiae*
ASO	antistreptolysin O
AST	aspartate aminotransferase
ATLL	adult T-cell leukemia/lymphoma
ATPase	adenosine triphosphatase
AV	arteriovenous, atrioventricular
AZT	azidothymidine (zidovudine)
BAL	British antilewisite (dimercaprol)
BCG	bacille Calmette–Guérin
BE	barium enema
BP	blood pressure
BPH	benign prostatic hypertrophy
BUN	blood urea nitrogen
CABG	coronary artery bypass grafting
CAD	coronary artery disease
CaEDTA	calcium edetate
CALLA	common acute lymphoblastic leukemia antigen
cAMP	cyclic adenosine monophosphate
C-ANCA	cytoplasmic antineutrophil cytoplasmic antibody
CBC	complete blood count
CBD	common bile duct
CCU	cardiac care unit
CD	cluster of differentiation
2-CdA	2-chlorodeoxyadenosine
CEA	carcinoembryonic antigen
CFTR	cystic fibrosis transmembrane conductance regulator
cGMP	cyclic guanosine monophosphate
CHF	congestive heart failure
CK	creatine kinase
CK-MB	creatine kinase, MB fraction
CLL	chronic lymphocytic leukemia
CML	chronic myelogenous leukemia
CMV	cytomegalovirus
CN	cranial nerve
CNS	central nervous system
COPD	chronic obstructive pulmonary disease
COX	cyclooxygenase
CP	cerebellopontine
CPAP	continuous positive airway pressure
CPK	creatine phosphokinase
CPPD	calcium pyrophosphate dihydrate
CPR	cardiopulmonary resuscitation
CREST	calcinosis, Raynaud phenomenon, esophageal involvement, sclerodactyly, telangiectasia (syndrome)
CRP	C-reactive protein
CSF	cerebrospinal fluid
CSOM	chronic suppurative otitis media
CT	cardiac transplant, computed tomography

CVA	cerebrovascular accident
CXR	chest x-ray
d4T	didehydrodeoxythymidine (stavudine)
DCS	decompression sickness
DDH	developmental dysplasia of the hip
ddI	dideoxyinosine (didanosine)
DES	diethylstilbestrol
DEXA	dual-energy x-ray absorptiometry
DHEAS	dehydroepiandrosterone sulfate
DIC	disseminated intravascular coagulation
DIF	direct immunofluorescence
DIP	distal interphalangeal (joint)
DKA	diabetic ketoacidosis
DL_{CO}	diffusing capacity of carbon monoxide
DMSA	2,3-dimercaptosuccinic acid
DNA	deoxyribonucleic acid
DNase	deoxyribonuclease
2,3-DPG	2,3-diphosphoglycerate
dsDNA	double-stranded DNA
DSM	Diagnostic and Statistical Manual
dsRNA	double-stranded RNA
DTP	diphtheria, tetanus, pertussis (vaccine)
DTPA	diethylenetriamine-penta-acetic acid
DTs	delirium tremens
DVT	deep venous thrombosis
EBV	Epstein–Barr virus
ECG	electrocardiography
Echo	echocardiography
ECM	erythema chronicum migrans
ECT	electroconvulsive therapy
EEG	electroencephalography
EF	ejection fraction, elongation factor
EGD	esophagogastroduodenoscopy
EHEC	enterohemorrhagic *Escherichia coli*
EIA	enzyme immunoassay
ELISA	enzyme-linked immunosorbent assay
EM	electron microscopy
EMG	electromyography
ENT	ears, nose, and throat
EPVE	early prosthetic valve endocarditis
ER	emergency room
ERCP	endoscopic retrograde cholangiopancreatography
ERT	estrogen replacement therapy
ESR	erythrocyte sedimentation rate
ETEC	enterotoxigenic *Escherichia coli*
EtOH	ethanol
FAP	familial adenomatous polyposis
FEV_1	forced expiratory volume in 1 second
FH	familial hypercholesterolemia
FNA	fine-needle aspiration
FSH	follicle-stimulating hormone
FTA-ABS	fluorescent treponemal antibody absorption test
FVC	forced vital capacity
G6PD	glucose-6-phosphate dehydrogenase
GABA	gamma-aminobutyric acid
GERD	gastroesophageal reflux disease
GFR	glomerular filtration rate
GGT	gamma-glutamyltransferase
GH	growth hormone
GI	gastrointestinal
GnRH	gonadotropin-releasing hormone
GU	genitourinary
GVHD	graft-versus-host disease
HAART	highly active antiretroviral therapy
HAV	hepatitis A virus
Hb	hemoglobin
HbA-1C	hemoglobin A-1C
HBsAg	hepatitis B surface antigen
HBV	hepatitis B virus
hCG	human chorionic gonadotropin
HCO_3	bicarbonate
Hct	hematocrit
HCV	hepatitis C virus
HDL	high-density lipoprotein
HDL-C	high-density lipoprotein-cholesterol
HEENT	head, eyes, ears, nose, and throat (exam)
HELLP	hemolysis, elevated LFTs, low platelets (syndrome)
HFMD	hand, foot, and mouth disease
HGPRT	hypoxanthine-guanine phosphoribosyltransferase
5-HIAA	5-hydroxyindoleacetic acid
HIDA	hepato-iminodiacetic acid (scan)

HIV	human immunodeficiency virus
HLA	human leukocyte antigen
HMG-CoA	hydroxymethylglutaryl-coenzyme A
HMP	hexose monophosphate
HPI	history of present illness
HPV	human papillomavirus
HR	heart rate
HRIG	human rabies immune globulin
HRS	hepatorenal syndrome
HRT	hormone replacement therapy
HSG	hysterosalpingography
HSV	herpes simplex virus
HTLV	human T-cell leukemia virus
HUS	hemolytic-uremic syndrome
HVA	homovanillic acid
ICP	intracranial pressure
ICU	intensive care unit
ID/CC	identification and chief complaint
IDDM	insulin-dependent diabetes mellitus
IFA	immunofluorescent antibody
Ig	immunoglobulin
IGF	insulin-like growth factor
IHSS	idiopathic hypertrophic subaortic stenosis
IM	intramuscular
IMA	inferior mesenteric artery
INH	isoniazid
INR	International Normalized Ratio
IP_3	inositol 1,4,5-triphosphate
IPF	idiopathic pulmonary fibrosis
ITP	idiopathic thrombocytopenic purpura
IUD	intrauterine device
IV	intravenous
IVC	inferior vena cava
IVIG	intravenous immunoglobulin
IVP	intravenous pyelography
JRA	juvenile rheumatoid arthritis
JVP	jugular venous pressure
KOH	potassium hydroxide
KUB	kidney, ureter, bladder
LCM	lymphocytic choriomeningitis
LDH	lactate dehydrogenase
LDL	low-density lipoprotein
LE	lupus erythematosus (cell)
LES	lower esophageal sphincter
LFTs	liver function tests
LH	luteinizing hormone
LMN	lower motor neuron
LP	lumbar puncture
LPVE	late prosthetic valve endocarditis
L/S	lecithin/sphingomyelin (ratio)
LSD	lysergic acid diethylamide
LT	labile toxin
LV	left ventricular
LVH	left ventricular hypertrophy
Lytes	electrolytes
Mammo	mammography
MAO	monoamine oxidase (inhibitor)
MCP	metacarpophalangeal (joint)
MCTD	mixed connective tissue disorder
MCV	mean corpuscular volume
MEN	multiple endocrine neoplasia
MI	myocardial infarction
MIBG	meta-iodobenzylguanidine (radioisotope)
MMR	measles, mumps, rubella (vaccine)
MPGN	membranoproliferative glomerulonephritis
MPS	mucopolysaccharide
MPTP	1-methyl-4-phenyl-tetrahydropyridine
MR	magnetic resonance (imaging)
mRNA	messenger ribonucleic acid
MRSA	methicillin-resistant *S. aureus*
MTP	metatarsophalangeal (joint)
NAD	nicotinamide adenine dinucleotide
NADP	nicotinamide adenine dinucleotide phosphate
NADPH	reduced nicotinamide adenine dinucleotide phosphate
NF	neurofibromatosis
NIDDM	non-insulin-dependent diabetes mellitus
NNRTI	non-nucleoside reverse transcriptase inhibitor
NO	nitric oxide
NPO	nil per os (nothing by mouth)
NSAID	nonsteroidal anti-inflammatory drug
Nuc	nuclear medicine
NYHA	New York Heart Association
OB	obstetric
OCD	obsessive–compulsive disorder
OCPs	oral contraceptive pills
OR	operating room

PA	posteroanterior
PABA	para-aminobenzoic acid
PAN	polyarteritis nodosa
P-ANCA	perinuclear antineutrophil cytoplasmic antibody
Pa_{O_2}	partial pressure of oxygen in arterial blood
PAS	periodic acid Schiff
PAT	paroxysmal atrial tachycardia
PBS	peripheral blood smear
Pc_{O_2}	partial pressure of carbon dioxide
PCOM	posterior communicating (artery)
PCOS	polycystic ovarian syndrome
PCP	phencyclidine
PCR	polymerase chain reaction
PCT	porphyria cutanea tarda
PCTA	percutaneous coronary transluminal angioplasty
PCV	polycythemia vera
PDA	patent ductus arteriosus
PDGF	platelet-derived growth factor
PE	physical exam
PEFR	peak expiratory flow rate
PEG	polyethylene glycol
PEPCK	phosphoenolpyruvate carboxykinase
PET	positron emission tomography
PFTs	pulmonary function tests
PID	pelvic inflammatory disease
PIP	proximal interphalangeal (joint)
PKU	phenylketonuria
PMDD	premenstrual dysphoric disorder
PML	progressive multifocal leukoencephalopathy
PMN	polymorphonuclear (leukocyte)
PNET	primitive neuroectodermal tumor
PNH	paroxysmal nocturnal hemoglobinuria
P_{O_2}	partial pressure of oxygen
PPD	purified protein derivative (of tuberculosis)
PPH	primary postpartum hemorrhage
PRA	panel reactive antibody
PROM	premature rupture of membranes
PSA	prostate-specific antigen
PSS	progressive systemic sclerosis
PT	prothrombin time
PTH	parathyroid hormone
PTSD	posttraumatic stress disorder
PTT	partial thromboplastin time
PUVA	psoralen ultraviolet A
PVC	premature ventricular contraction
RA	rheumatoid arthritis
RAIU	radioactive iodine uptake
RAST	radioallergosorbent test
RBC	red blood cell
REM	rapid eye movement
RES	reticuloendothelial system
RFFIT	rapid fluorescent focus inhibition test
RFTs	renal function tests
RHD	rheumatic heart disease
RNA	ribonucleic acid
RNP	ribonucleoprotein
RPR	rapid plasma reagin
RR	respiratory rate
RSV	respiratory syncytial virus
RUQ	right upper quadrant
RV	residual volume
Sa_{O_2}	oxygen saturation in arterial blood
SBFT	small bowel follow-through
SCC	squamous cell carcinoma
SCID	severe combined immunodeficiency
SERM	selective estrogen receptor modulator
SGOT	serum glutamic-oxaloacetic transaminase
SIADH	syndrome of inappropriate antidiuretic hormone
SIDS	sudden infant death syndrome
SLE	systemic lupus erythematosus
SMA	superior mesenteric artery
SSPE	subacute sclerosing panencephalitis
SSRI	selective serotonin-reuptake inhibitor
ST	stable toxin
STD	sexually transmitted disease
T2W	T2-weighted (MRI)
T_3	triiodothyronine
T_4	thyroxine
TAH-BSO	total abdominal hysterectomy–bilateral salpingo-oophorectomy

TB tuberculosis
TCA tricyclic antidepressant
TCC transitional cell carcinoma
TDT terminal deoxytransferase
TFTs thyroid function tests
TGF transforming growth factor
THC tetrahydrocannabinol
TIA transient ischemic attack
TLC total lung capacity
TMP-SMX trimethoprim-sulfamethoxazole
tPA tissue plasminogen activator
TP-HA *Treponema pallidum* hemagglutination assay
TPP thiamine pyrophosphate
TRAP tartrate-resistant acid phosphatase
tRNA transfer ribonucleic acid
TSH thyroid-stimulating hormone
TSS toxic shock syndrome
TTP thrombotic thrombocytopenic purpura
TURP transurethral resection of the prostate
TXA thromboxane A
UA urinalysis
UDCA ursodeoxycholic acid
UGI upper GI
UPPP uvulopalatopharyngoplasty
URI upper respiratory infection
US ultrasound
UTI urinary tract infection
UV ultraviolet
VDRL Venereal Disease Research Laboratory
VIN vulvar intraepithelial neoplasia
VIP vasoactive intestinal polypeptide
VLDL very low density lipoprotein
VMA vanillylmandelic acid
V/Q ventilation/perfusion (ratio)
VRE vancomycin-resistant enterococcus
VS vital signs
VSD ventricular septal defect
vWF von Willebrand factor
VZV varicella-zoster virus
WAGR Wilms tumor, aniridia, genitourinary abnormalities, mental retardation (syndrome)
WBC white blood cell
WHI Women's Health Initiative
WPW Wolff–Parkinson–White syndrome
XR x-ray
ZN Ziehl–Neelsen (stain)

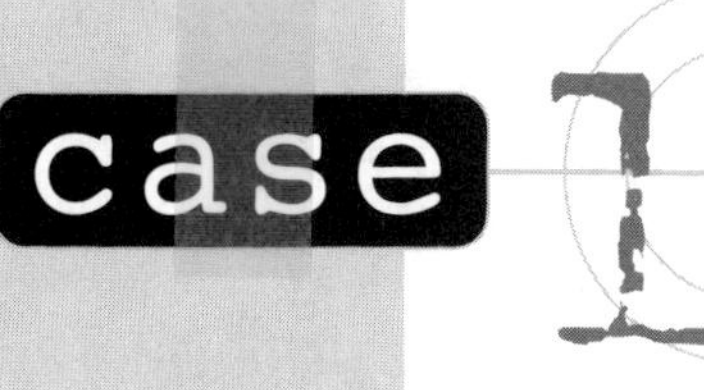

case 1

ID/CC A 48-year-old **man** with a history of **hypertension** is brought by ambulance to the emergency room because of the development of **sudden sharp, tearing, intractable left chest pain with radiation to the back.**

HPI When he first arrives, he shows a declining level of consciousness, becomes **pale** and **short of breath** (DYSPNEA), has **decreased urine output** (OLIGURIA), and is unable to move his left arm and leg; subsequently he **faints** (SYNCOPE).

PE VS: **marked hypotension** (BP 90/50) in left arm, with significantly higher reading in right arm (BP 170/80). PE: **pallor; cyanosis; diaphoresis;** indistinct heart sounds; **aortic regurgitation murmur** (high-pitched, blowing, diastolic decrescendo murmur); inspiratory crackles at lung bases bilaterally (due to pulmonary edema); **anuria** (due to decreased renal perfusion); **left-sided hemiplegia.**

Labs ECG: no evidence of myocardial infarct.

Imaging CT/MR: **spiraling intimal flap with true and false lumen** (DOUBLE-BARREL AORTA). Angio, aortography: confirmatory. CXR: **mediastinal widening** (due to hemorrhage).

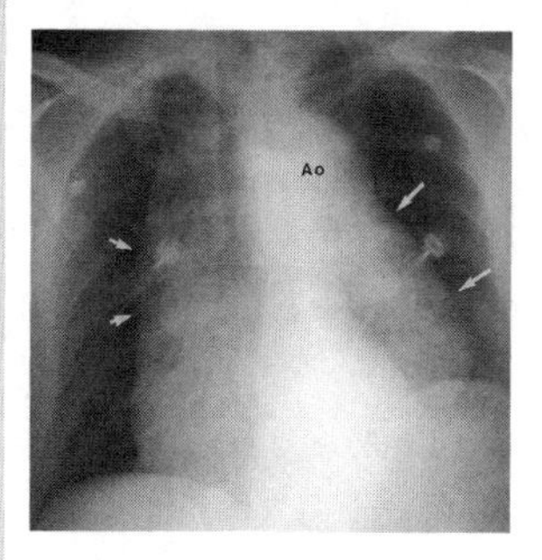

Figure 1-1. Posteroanterior chest examination shows marked widening of the mediastinum.

Gross Pathology Longitudinal separation of tunica media of aortic wall.

case 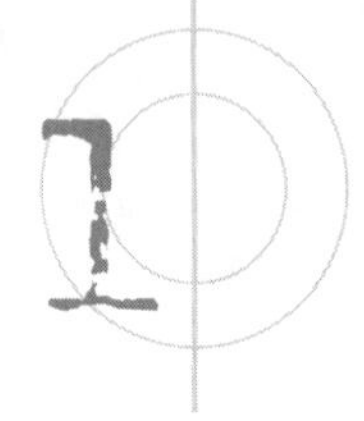

Aortic Dissection

Differential

Myocardial infarction
Pancreatitis
Cardiac tamponade
Pulmonary embolism
Myocarditis
Hypovolemic shock

Discussion

Aortic dissection is a **life-threatening** condition requiring immediate treatment. Predisposing factors include **hypertension** and connective tissue diseases (cystic medial degeneration as in Marfan syndrome); complications include rupture and extension. **Sudden death** may occur with **pericardial tamponade** or **extension of dissection into coronary arteries.**

Treatment

ICU monitoring for shock; antihypertensive agents (preferably beta-blockers) to decrease vascular shear forces (avoid arteriolar dilators such as hydralazine); surgical correction.

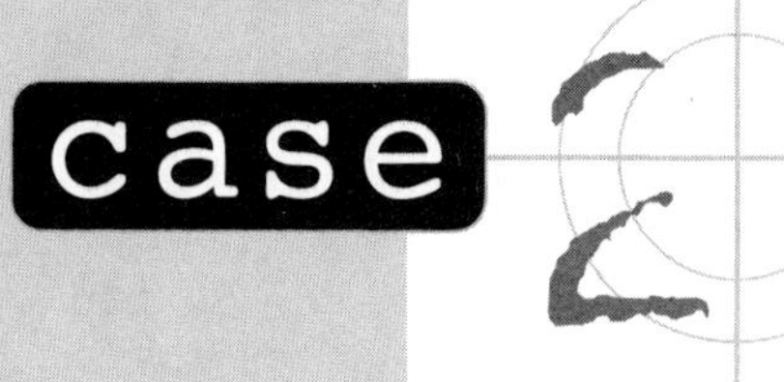

ID/CC A 31-year-old white man who was diagnosed with **Marfan syndrome** more than 20 years ago **recently** developed **severe shortness of breath.**

HPI He denies smoking or drinking and claims to have had no major illnesses in the past.

PE VS: **pulse bounding, large in volume, and collapsing** (WATER-HAMMER OR CORRIGAN PULSE), producing **wide pulse pressure** with rapid rise and fall. PE: soft, high-pitched, blowing **diastolic decrescendo murmur heard best at left sternal border** with patient leaning forward and in expiration; diastolic murmur heard when femoral artery compressed with stethoscope (DUROZIEZ SIGN).

Labs ECG: left ventricular hypertrophy (LVH).

Imaging CXR: left ventricular dilatation. Echo: LVH; Doppler confirmatory.

Gross Pathology Caused by defect of aortic valves or roots that leads to regurgitation of blood from aorta into left ventricle.

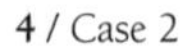

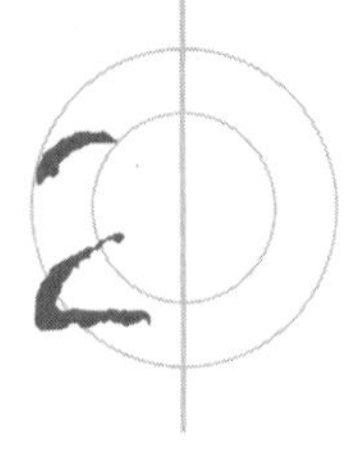

case 2

Aortic Insufficiency

Differential

Mitral stenosis
Pulmonary regurgitation
Tricuspid stenosis
Ventricular septal defect

Discussion

Common causes of aortic insufficiency include congenital bicuspid valve and infective endocarditis; less common causes include rheumatic heart disease and aortic root diseases (e.g., Marfan syndrome, ankylosing spondylitis, Reiter syndrome, tertiary syphilis).

Treatment

Surgical **prosthetic valve replacement** for symptomatic patients or for asymptomatic patients with LV dysfunction. For symptomatic patients with normal LV function, diuretics or afterload-reducing drugs may be beneficial. Antibiotic prophylaxis against infective endocarditis before undergoing surgical or dental procedures.

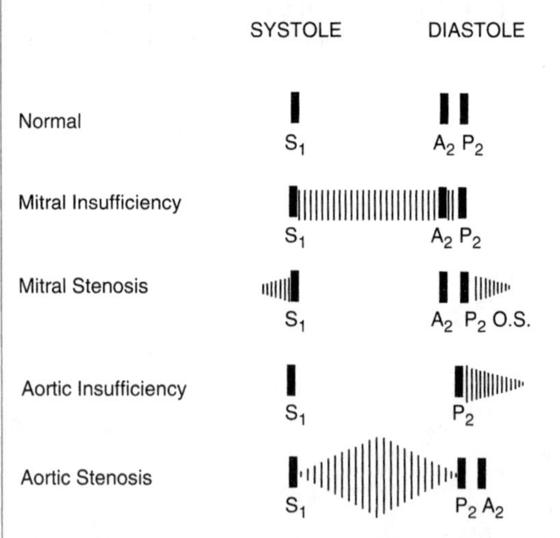

Figure 2-1. The position of heart sounds and murmurs in several valvular lesions.

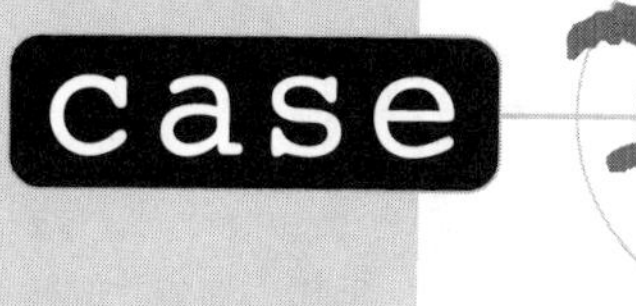

ID/CC A **24-year-old** man complains of easy fatigability, dyspnea on mild exertion, and **angina.**

HPI He also admits to having occasional spells of **lightheadedness** and **fainting** while playing basketball.

PE **Crescendo–decrescendo systolic ejection murmur to right of sternum and radiating to neck;** soft S2 with **paradoxical splitting** (due to pulmonary valve closure preceding aortic valve closure); weak and delayed ("parvus et tardus") carotid pulses.

Labs ECG: left ventricular hypertrophy.

Imaging CXR: calcifications on valve leaflets and enlarged cardiac shadow (due to large left ventricle). Echo: presence of bicuspid aortic valve.

Gross Pathology Congenital bicuspid valve with calcification.

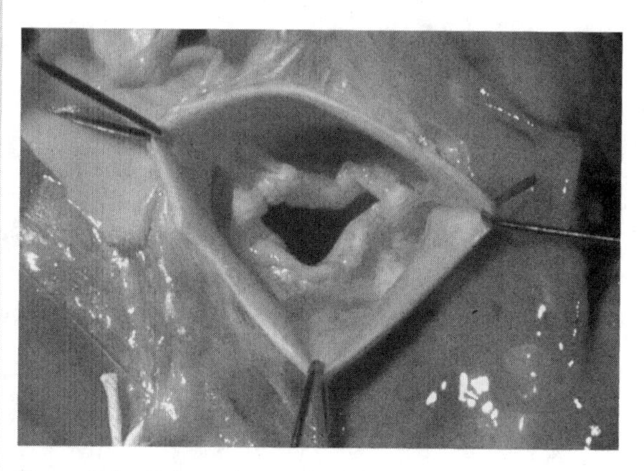

Figure 3-1. Deformation and calcium deposition of the aortic valve cusps.

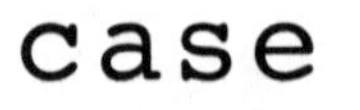
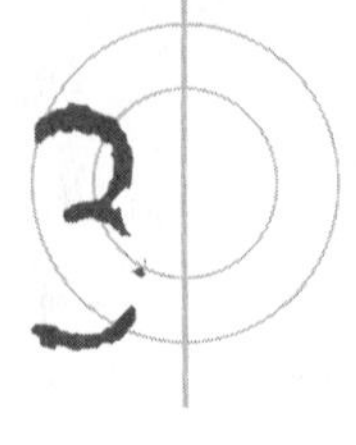

Aortic Stenosis

Differential

Mitral regurgitation
Mitral valve prolapse
Hypertrophic obstructive cardiomyopathy
Myocardial infarction

Discussion

Causes of aortic stenosis include **congenital bicuspid aortic valve** (more common in men), **progressive degenerative calcification** of normal valves (more common in older men), and rheumatic heart disease (the mitral valve is also involved in 95% of individuals with rheumatic disease of the aortic valve).

Treatment

Balloon valvuloplasty; surgical aortic valve replacement; antibiotic prophylaxis with penicillin prior to surgical or dental procedures.

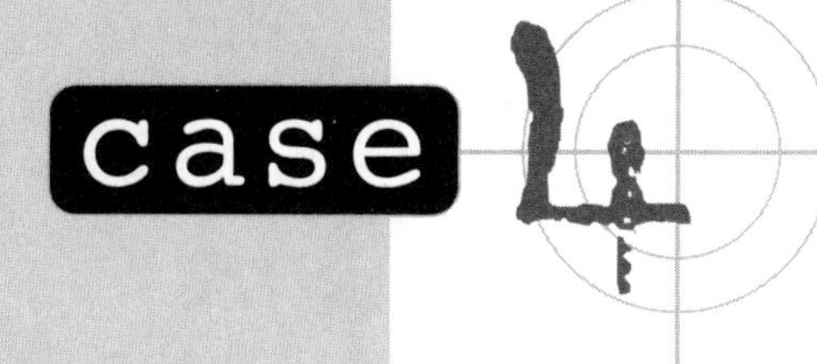

ID/CC A 59-year-old white man complains of **pain in the calf muscles** during exercise (CLAUDICATION) along with coldness and numbness in both legs; his symptoms have been occurring for a year and are **relieved by rest.**

HPI The patient has also been **impotent** and has been experiencing abdominal pain (due to mesenteric ischemia) about half an hour after eating (POSTPRANDIAL PAIN). He **smokes** two packs of cigarettes a day.

PE VS: **hypertension** (BP 150/100). PE: **diminished peripheral pulses** bilaterally; **loss of hair** over dorsum of feet and hands; decreased temperature in hands and feet; **carotid and femoral arterial bruits**; atrophy of calf muscles.

Labs **Elevated LDL and decreased HDL;** elevated total serum cholesterol.

Imaging Angio: multiple large **atheromatous plaques in aortoiliac distribution.** XR, plain: irregular arterial vascular calcifications. US, Doppler: high-velocity poststenotic flow jet.

Gross Pathology Early: fatty streak in subendothelium; late: **fibrofatty plaque** formation with dystrophic calcification (atheroma) with narrowing of lumen of vessel wall.

Micro Pathology Early: **foam cells** with intimal proliferation of smooth muscle cells; late: smooth muscle cells synthesize collagen and form **fibrous cap** with **necrotic lipid core** and fibrous plaque.

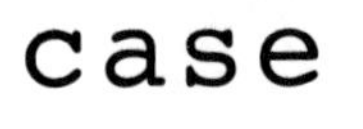
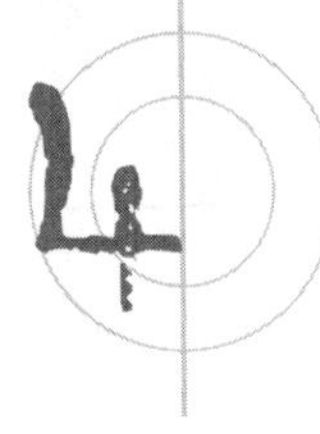

case 4

Atherosclerosis

Differential

Diabetic neuropathy
Vasculitis
Collagen vascular disease
Familial hypercholesterolemia

Discussion

Atherosclerosis is the main cause of coronary artery disease and the leading cause of mortality in the United States. Plaques are commonly found in the abdominal aorta, coronary arteries, popliteal arteries, descending thoracic aorta, internal carotid arteries, and circle of Willis arteries. Thus, they are responsible for aortic aneurysms, CAD, peripheral vascular disease, intestinal angina, renovascular hypertension, and cerebrovascular disease.

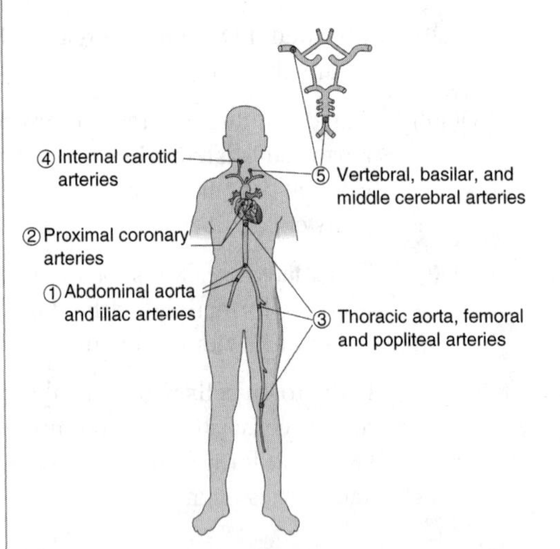

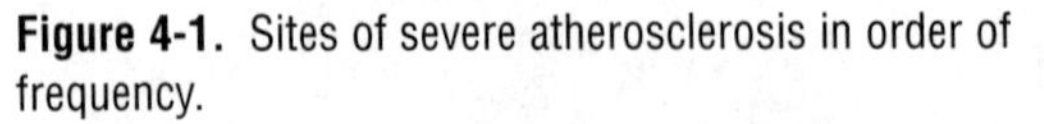
Figure 4-1. Sites of severe atherosclerosis in order of frequency.

Treatment

Exercise; dietary modifications; smoking cessation; low-dose aspirin; control of hypertension; cholesterol-lowering drugs (e.g., lovastatin); angioplasty; coronary stenting; coronary artery bypass grafting (CABG).

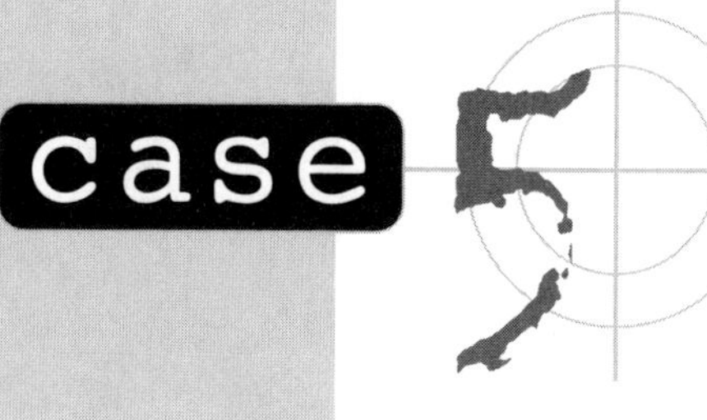

ID/CC A 47-year-old man complains of occasional **palpitations** and **shortness of breath.**

HPI He also says that he occasionally experiences mild **dizziness** and chest discomfort.

PE VS: **irregularly irregular** pulse. PE: loss of a waves in jugular venous pulse; variable-intensity S1 with occasional S3.

Labs ECG: variable ventricular rate (80 to 200); can be >200 with wide QRS if associated with accessory pathway; **Irregular RR intervals.** Normal CK-MB.

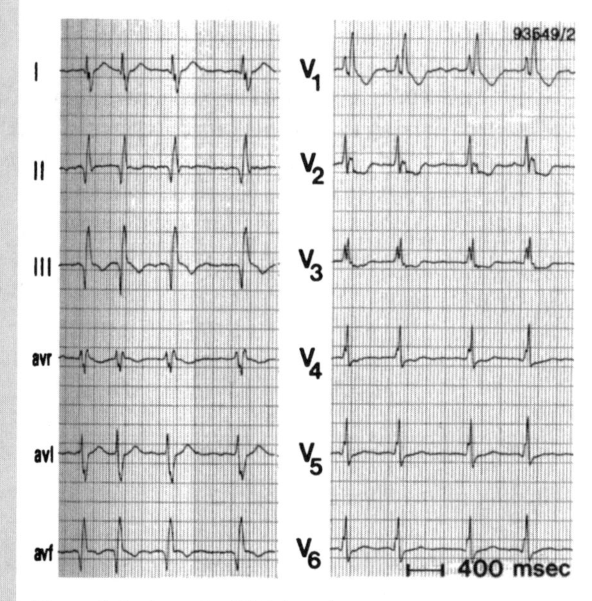

Figure 5-1. Irregular RR intervals.

Imaging CXR: normal. Echo: enlarged left atrium.

case 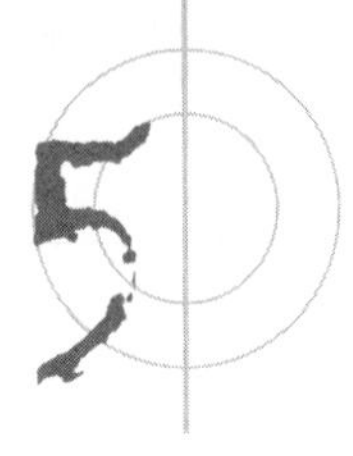

Atrial Fibrillation

Differential

Atrial flutter

Atrial tachycardia

Paroxysmal supraventricular tachycardia

Wolff–Parkinson–White syndrome

Discussion

Atrial fibrillation, the most common chronic arrhythmia, is associated with a high risk of **embolic disease.** Causes include drugs, mitral valve disease, hypertensive and ischemic heart disease, dilated cardiomyopathy, alcoholism, **hyperthyroidism**, pericarditis, pulmonary embolism, exercise, atrial septal defect, chronic lung disease, and cardiac surgery. It may also be idiopathic.

Treatment

Beta-blockers; calcium channel blockers; digitalis (to decrease conduction at AV node in order to control ventricular rate; chemical cardioversion with **class IA, IC, or III antiarrhythmics** to convert back to sinus rhythm if patient remains symptomatic; **electrical cardioversion**; patients should also be **anticoagulated** with warfarin to prevent embolic disease.

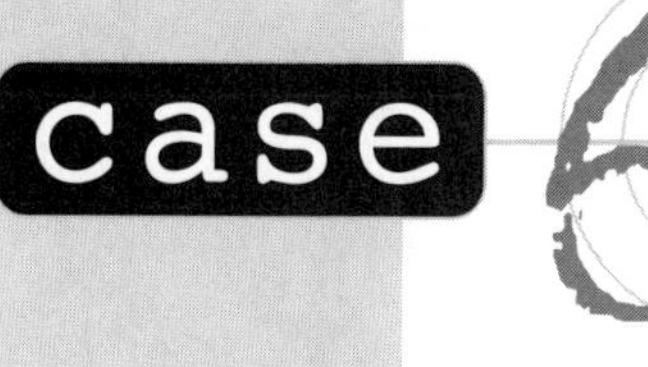

ID/CC A **50-year-old woman** complains of recurrent, **transient losses of consciousness** (SYNCOPE) and **dizziness.**

HPI For the past few months she has had continuous mild to moderate **fever, fatigue, sweating, and joint pains** (ARTHRALGIAS) and has experienced unexplainable **breathlessness at rest** (episodic pulmonary edema) that is **relieved in a supine position and exacerbated by standing.** She also complains of significant **weight loss** over the past year.

PE VS: **mild fever.** PE: pallor and clubbing; on auscultation, **S1 delayed and decreased in intensity** and characteristic **low-pitched sound during early diastole,** followed by a rumble; **auscultatory findings vary with body position.**

Labs CBC: normochromic, normocytic anemia. **Elevated ESR;** increased IgG; blood cultures sterile. ECG: **sinus rhythm.**

Imaging Echo (2D): characteristic echo-producing **mass in left atrium.** MR, cardiac: globular **mass** in left atrium.

Gross Pathology Single globular left atrial mass about 6 cm in diameter, pedunculated with fibrovascular stalk arising from **interatrial septum** in vicinity of **fossa ovalis** (favored site of atrial origin).

Micro Pathology **Stellate, multipotential mesenchymal cells** mixed with **endothelial cells;** mature and immature smooth muscle cells and macrophages, all in an **acid mucopolysaccharide matrix.**

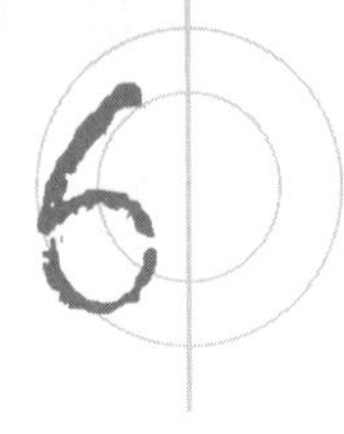

case 6

Atrial Myxoma

Differential

Mitral regurgitation
Mitral stenosis
Carcinoid heart disease
Left atrial thrombus

Discussion

The **most common type of primary cardiac tumors,** myxomas, may be located in any of the four chambers or, rarely, in the valves. They are **predominantly atrial with a 4:1 left-to-right ratio** and are **usually single.** Their signs and symptoms are closely related to their location and to the patient's position. Although myxomas are benign, they can embolize, resulting in metastatic disease. Although most myxomas are sporadic, some are familial with **autosomal dominant** transmission; thus, echocardiographic **screening** of first-degree relatives is appropriate.

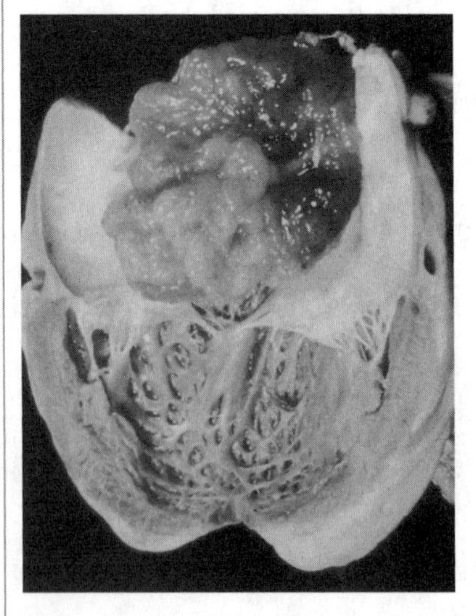

Figure 6-1. Cardiac myxoma.

Treatment

Surgical excision using cardiopulmonary bypass is curative.

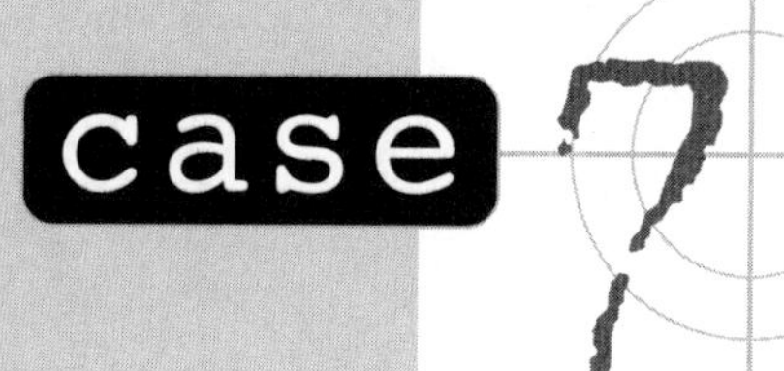

ID/CC A **78-year-old** white **man** is brought into the ER with **nausea, dyspnea,** and a **crushing substernal chest pain** that **radiates to** his **left arm and jaw;** the pain has lasted for about 30 minutes and is not relieved with rest.

HPI One sublingual nitroglycerin tablet did not relieve his pain. His history reveals a **sedentary lifestyle, moderate hypercholesterolemia,** and **obesity.** The patient is also has **diabetes** and **smokes.**

PE VS: hypotension. PE: **diaphoresis.**

Labs ECG: **ST elevation** with peaking of T waves; subsequent development of **inverted T waves** and **permanent Q waves.** Later, ST and T waves normalize. **Elevated CK-MB; elevated troponin T and I.** CBC: leukocytosis.

Imaging Echo: **decreased wall motion** (HYPOKINESIS).

Gross Pathology 12 hours: no myocardial damage; 24 hours: pallor due to coagulation necrosis or reddish mottling; 3 to 5 days: demarcated yellow region with hyperemic border; 2 to 3 weeks: soft, gelatinous; 1 to 2 months: white scar and firm, thin wall.

Micro Pathology 12 to 18 hours: nuclear pyknosis, **coagulation necrosis,** and eosinophilia; 1 to 3 days: intense neutrophilic infiltrate, loss of nuclei and crossstriations; 1 week: disappearance of PMNs, onset of fibroblastic repair; 3 weeks: granulation tissue with progressive fibrosis.

case 7

CAD—Myocardial Infarction

Differential

Anxiety
Gastrointestinal reflux disease
Myocarditis
Pneumothorax
Pulmonary embolism

Discussion

The most common cause of myocardial infarction is atherosclerosis (coronary artery disease); it is less commonly caused by coronary vasospasm (Prinzmetal angina). Sequelae include arrhythmias, congestive heart failure, pulmonary edema, shock, pulmonary embolism, papillary muscle rupture, ventricular aneurysm, ventricular wall rupture, tamponade, and autoimmune fibrinous pericarditis (DRESSLER SYNDROME).

Treatment

Oxygen, bed rest, aspirin, pain relief with morphine, nitrates, beta-blockers; plaque stabilization with heparin, anti-Gp IIa-IIIb monoclonal antibodies; thrombolysis with tPA if cardiac catheterization is not immediately available; cardiac catheterization with angioplasty or surgical reperfusion with a bypass graft depending on nature of disease; ACE inhibitors (limit postinfarct remodeling) and cholesterol-lowering drugs.

Breakout Point

Treatment for myocardial infarction
MONA B:
- ***M***orphine
- ***O***xygen
- ***N***itroglycerine
- ***A***spirin
- ***B***eta-blocker

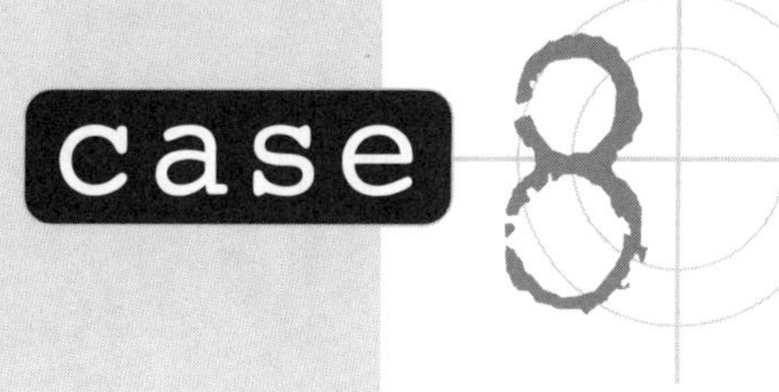

case 8

ID/CC A 50-year-old man who was admitted to the CCU **3 days ago** following an **MI** presents with **hypotension.**

HPI The patient was thrombolyzed post-MI and was recovering well. He also complained of a mild fever but no chills or rigors.

PE VS: tachycardia; weak, thready pulse; tachypnea; **hypotension.** PE: pallor; cool, moist skin; mild cyanosis of lips and digits; >10-mmHg fall in arterial pressure with inspiration (PULSUS PARADOXUS); **heart sounds muffled** and **JVP elevated;** lungs clear bilaterally.

Labs Elevated cardiac enzymes (CK-MB, troponin) as a result of recent acute MI.

Imaging Echo: diastolic compression of the right ventricle; pericardial effusion.

Gross Pathology Rupture of the left ventricular wall with hemopericardium.

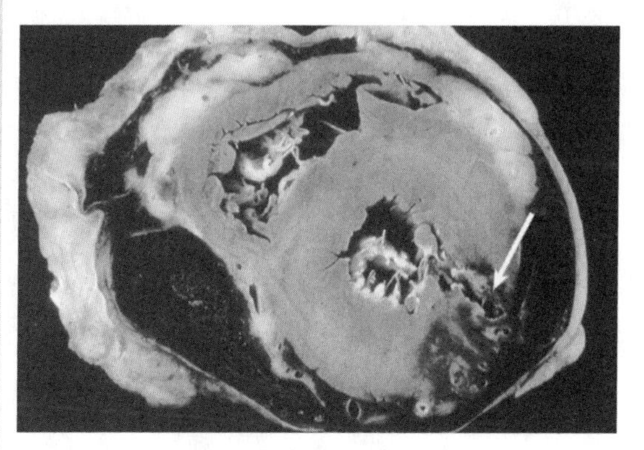

Figure 8-1. Rupture of a myocardial infarct (arrow) with accumulation of large quantities of blood in the pericardial cavity.

Micro Pathology Ischemic coagulative necrosis of the affected myocardium, consisting of multiple erythrocytes and dead, anucleated myocytes.

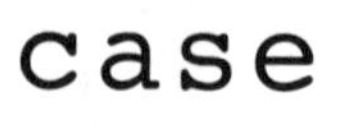
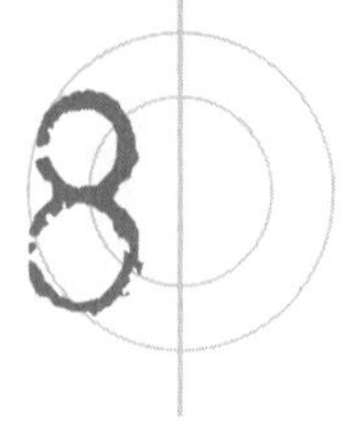

Cardiac Tamponade

Differential

Cardiogenic shock
Constrictive pericarditis
Pulmonary embolism
Tension pneumothorax

Discussion

Cardiac rupture most typically develops 3 to 10 days after the initial onset of the infarction secondary to rupture of necrotic cardiac muscle; there is usually little warning before the sudden collapse, which is associated with acute cardiac tamponade and electromechanical dissociation. Papillary muscle rupture may also occur following an acute MI, resulting in mitral regurgitation and left ventricular failure.

Treatment

Emergency pericardiocentesis; treat shock by infusing fluid and isoproterenol; surgical repair of cardiac rupture subsequent to stabilization.

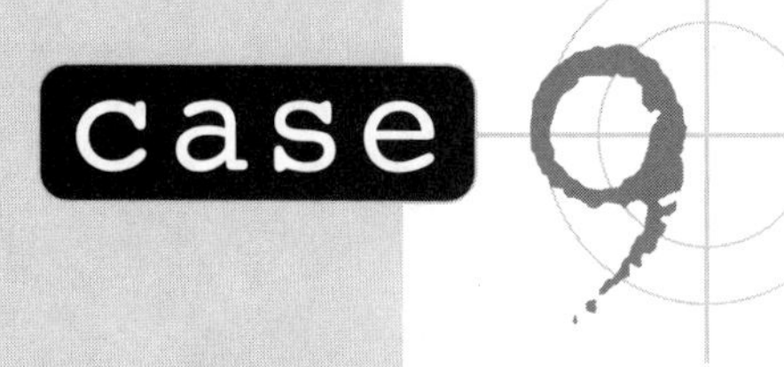

case 9

ID/CC A 60-year-old man presents to a clinic for a **heart transplant evaluation.**

HPI The patient was diagnosed last year with **class III** (marked limitation of activity; comfortable only at rest) **congestive heart failure** secondary to **idiopathic dilated cardiomyopathy.** He is currently being treated with digoxin, furosemide (diuretic), lisinopril (ACE inhibitor), and warfarin (anticoagulant) but continues to be symptomatic.

PE VS: normal. PE: elevated JVP; S3/S4 gallop heard on auscultation; significant pitting lower extremity **edema.**

Labs CBC/Lytes: Normal. TFTs, LFTs, total protein, albumin, uric acid, and 24-hour protein/creatinine normal; PSA normal; IgG and IgM antibody titers against CMV, HSV, HIV, VZV, hepatitis B and C, and toxoplasmosis negative; PT/PTT/INR normal.

Imaging Echo: EF 15% with moderate mitral valve regurgitation. CXR: **cardiomegaly.** ECG: occasional **premature ventricular contractions (PVCs).** Thallium scan: **exercise-induced global cardiac ischemia.**

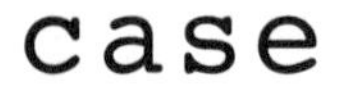

case 9

Cardiac Transplant

Discussion

Cardiac transplantation accounts for 14% of organ transplant procedures and can dramatically improve cardiac function in individuals with end-stage cardiac disease. Patients must have **New York Heart Association (NYHA) class III or IV congestive heart failure,** having failed maximum medical therapy and other therapeutic interventions such as PCTA for CAD. Currently, **ischemic heart disease** accounts for approximately 55% of causes requiring CT and **idiopathic cardiomyopathy** for roughly 40%.

Treatment

If approved as a viable transplant candidate, the patient must wait for a suitable donor (matched according to body size, weight, **ABO blood grouping,** and levels of **panel reactive antibody,** or **PRA**). A large number of patients waiting for a cardiac transplant (CT) die before a donor can be found.

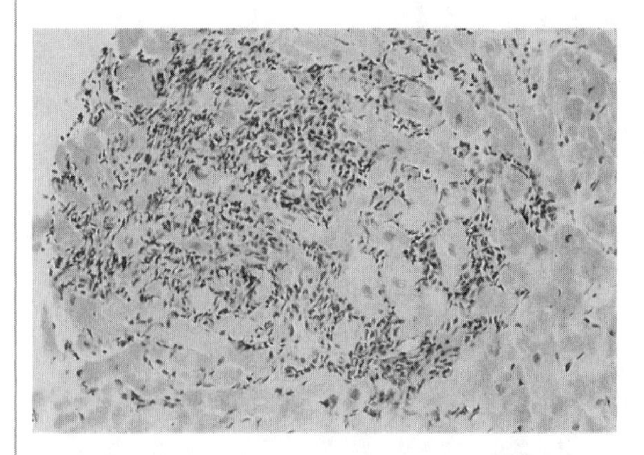

Figure 9-1. Microscopic consequences of cardiac transplant rejection: lymphocytic infiltration of mycocardium.

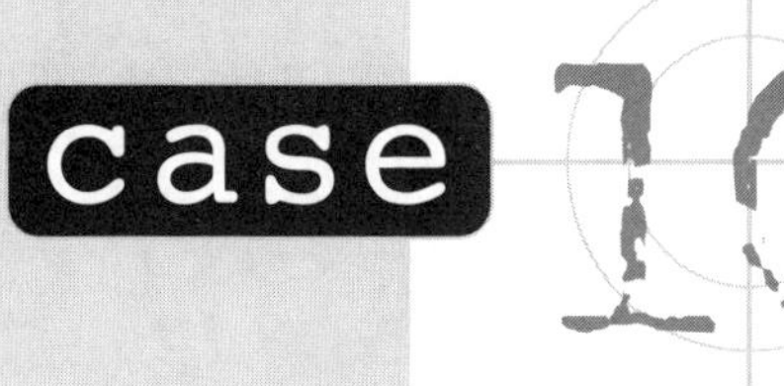

case 10

ID/CC A 65-year-old white man complains of **requiring three pillows in bed in order to breathe comfortably** (ORTHOPNEA) and having to open the window to **gasp for air at night** (PAROXYSMAL NOCTURNAL DYSPNEA).

HPI He has also noted **increasing shortness of breath** while walking as well as **swelling of his ankles and legs.** He had a **myocardial infarction** 2 years ago and has a history of **chronic hypertension.**

PE **Distention of neck veins** (due to elevated JVP); **third heart sound;** grade III/VI crescendo aortic systolic murmur; **crepitant rales** over both lower lobes; **lower lung fields dull to percussion** bilaterally; tender hepatomegaly; 4 **pitting edema** in both lower extremities; cold extremities.

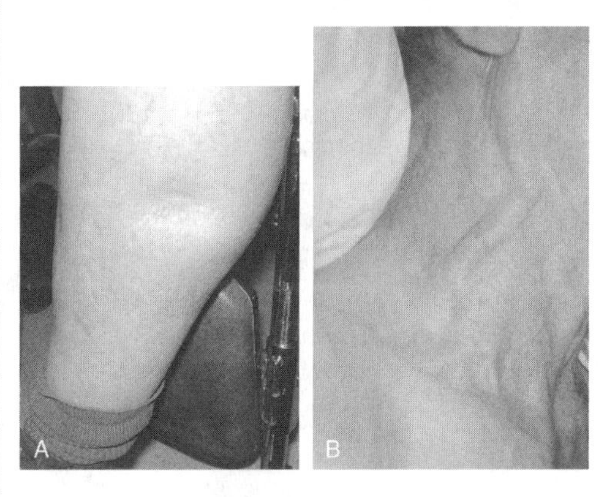

Figure 10-1. Pitting edema (A) and increased jugular venous distention (B).

Labs ABGs: hypoxemia; ECG: left ventricular hypertrophy.

Imaging CXR: enlarged cardiac silhouette; bilateral pleural effusions and diffuse increased lung markings (KERLEY B LINES) suggesting pulmonary edema.

Gross Pathology Cardiomegaly; pulmonary edema; **nutmeg liver** (due to chronic passive congestion).

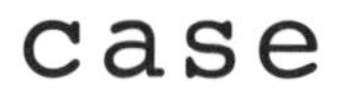
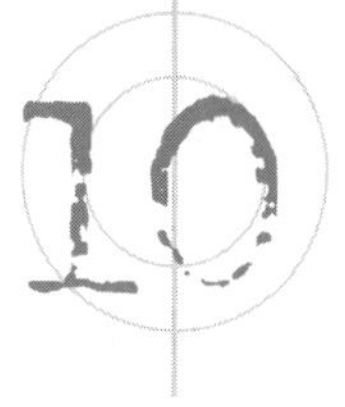

Congestive Heart Failure

Differential

Mitral regurgitation
Mitral valve prolapse
Hypertrophic obstructive cardiomyopathy
Myocardial infarction

Discussion

Congestive heart failure (CHF) is heart failure due to a deficit in myocardial strength or to an increase in workload. CHF is a common complication of ischemic and hypertensive heart disease in older populations. Can be classified according to severity based on the New York Heart Association (NYHA) classification

TABLE 10-1 NYHA CLASSIFICATIONS

Functional Assessment
Class I
No limitation of physical activity; ordinary physical activity does not cause undue dyspnea or fatigue, chest pain, or near syncope
Class II
Slight limitation of physical activity; comfortable at rest; ordinary physical activity causes undue dyspnea or fatigue, chest pain, or near syncope
Class III
Marked limitation of physical activity; comfortable at rest; less than ordinary activity causes undue dyspnea or fatigue, chest pain, or near syncope
Class IV
Unable to carry out any physical activity without symptoms; dyspnea and/or fatigue may be present at rest; discomfort is increased by any physical activity; signs of right heart failure are present

Treatment

Diuretics; low-sodium diet, digoxin; ACE inhibitors; nitrates; antiarrhythmics.

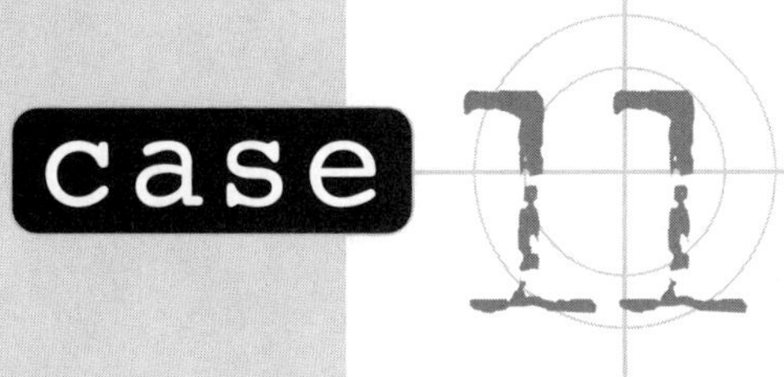

case 11

ID/CC A 35-year-old woman who is an **Asian** immigrant complains of weakness, **shortness of breath on exertion,** and **swelling of both feet.**

HPI She also complains of **progressive abdominal distension** and fatigue. She was treated for **pulmonary tuberculosis** a few years ago.

PE VS: mild hypotension; **reduced pulse pressure.** PE: peripheral cyanosis and cold extremities; pallor; neck veins distended; **JVP increases during inspiration** (KUSSMAUL SIGN); pedal edema; moderate hepatomegaly, splenomegaly, and ascites; **reduced-intensity apical impulse, distant heart sounds, and early third heart sound (pericardial knock).**

Labs ECG: **low-voltage** QRS complexes with flattening of T wave (nonspecific). LFTs mildly abnormal (due to hepatic congestion); ascitic fluid **transudative.**

Imaging CXR: **fibrosis** (old healed tuberculosis); heart shadow shows signs of **pericardial calcification.** Echo: **pericardial thickening.**

Gross Pathology Thick, dense, **fibrous obliteration of pericardial space with calcification.**

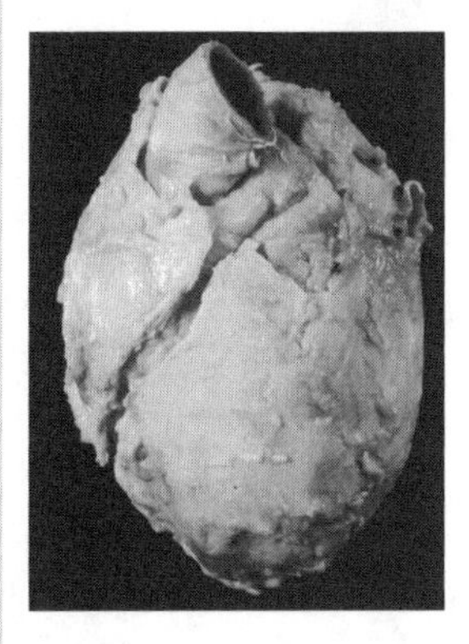

Figure 11-1. Obliteration of the pericardial space with encasement of the heart in a fibrotic, thickened pericardium.

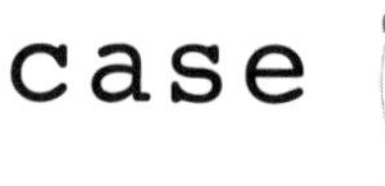

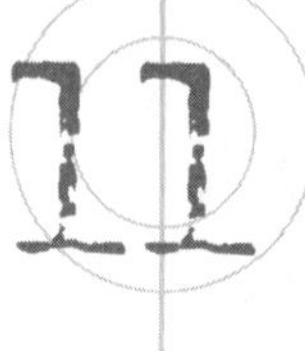

Constrictive Pericarditis

Differential

Atrial myxoma
Cardiac tamponade
Hemochromatosis
Nephrotic syndrome
Congestive heart failure

Discussion

The etiology of constrictive pericarditis lies in the formation of scar tissue that encases the heart and interferes with ventricular filling. **Tuberculosis** is the most common cause worldwide. Most cases now seen in the United States are idiopathic, but cases resulting from exposure to **radiation,** trauma, cardiac surgery, rheumatoid arthritis, or uremia have become more common.

Treatment

Complete pericardial resection is the only definitive treatment; institute **antituberculous therapy** when appropriate; diuretics; sodium restriction; digitalis for associated atrial fibrillation (in one third of patients).

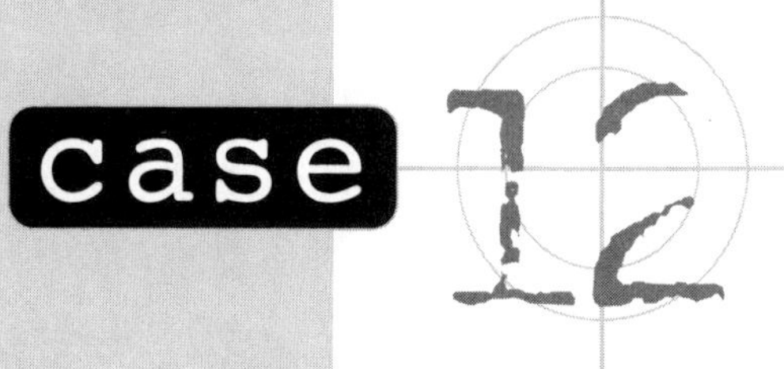

case 12

ID/CC A 60-year-old white man who has been treated for **COPD** comes to the emergency room with severe **dyspnea at rest.**

HPI Over the past few months, the patient has noted an **increased productive cough** and **exertional dyspnea.** He admits to being a **heavy smoker** and failed to quit smoking even after the appearance of **symptoms and the diagnosis of COPD.**

PE **Elevated JVP** with large a and v waves; **loud P2**; cyanosis; bilateral wheezing; expiratory rhonchi; prolonged expiration; use of accessory muscles of respiration; left parasternal heave; **ankle and sacral edema; tender hepatomegaly.**

Labs ECG: **right-axis deviation** and **peaked P waves** (P PULMONALE). PFTs: COPD pattern.

Imaging CXR: right ventricular and **pulmonary artery enlargement; hyperinflation.**

Gross Pathology Right ventricular hypertrophy.

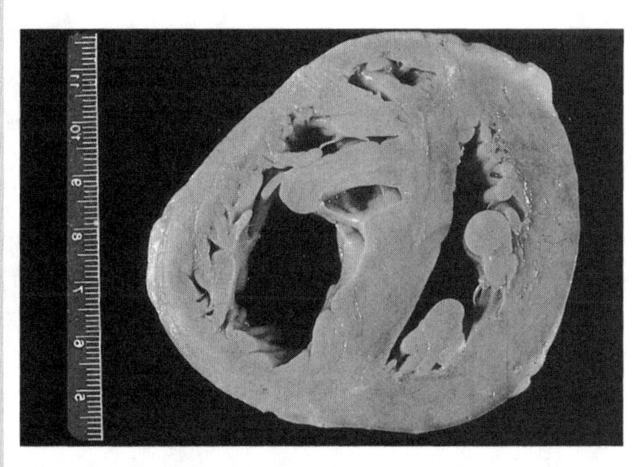

Figure 12-1. Marked hypertrophy of the right ventricle.

case 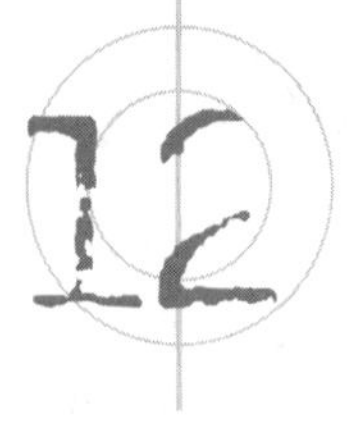

Cor Pulmonale

Differential

Ventricular septal defect
Congestive heart failure
Primary pulmonary hypertension
Right ventricular infarction

Discussion

Cor pulmonale is **right heart failure due to a pulmonary cause,** most commonly COPD. Other causes are pulmonary fibrosis, pneumoconiosis, recurrent pulmonary embolism, primary pulmonary hypertension, obesity with sleep apnea, cystic fibrosis, bronchiectasis, and kyphoscoliosis.

Treatment

Oxygen; salt and water restriction; treatment of COPD.

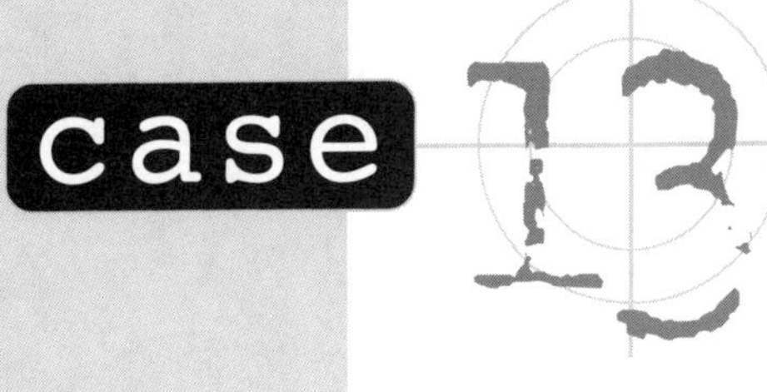

ID/CC A 29-year-old woman who **recently gave birth** to a healthy infant develops **dyspnea** and **swelling of her feet** toward the end of the day.

HPI She is nursing her 6-week-old child.

PE VS: BP mildly elevated. PE: JVP raised with prominent a and v waves; tender, mild hepatosplenomegaly; cardiac apex heaving and displaced outside midclavicular line; **pansystolic apical murmur** (due to **mitral insufficiency**) and systolic murmur increasing with inspiration heard in tricuspid area (due to tricuspid insufficiency); loud pulmonary component of S2; S3 and S4 gallop; fine inspiratory basal crepitant rales at both lung bases; pedal edema.

Labs ECG: premature ventricular contractions.

Imaging CXR: interstitial pulmonary edema (due to severe pulmonary venous hypertension); **global cardiomegaly.** Echo/Nuc: cardiomegaly with diminished ventricular contractility **(systolic dysfunction).** Stress test: **decreased ejection fraction with stress** (ejection fraction normally increases with stress).

Gross Pathology Global dilatation of all chambers.

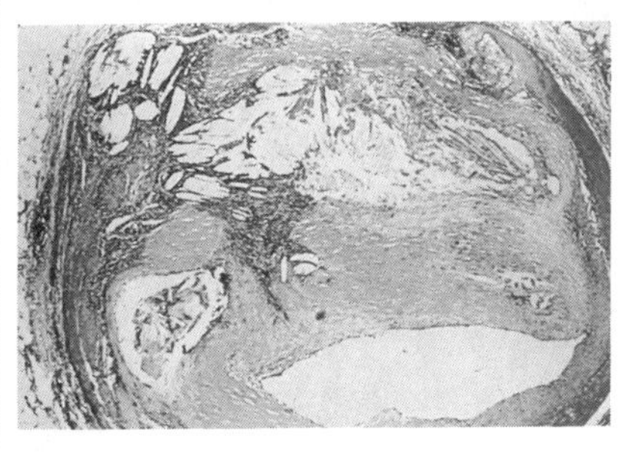

Figure 13-1. A transverse section of an enlarged heart reveals conspicuous dilation of both ventricles.

Micro Pathology **Extensive fibrosis without active inflammation** on endocardial biopsy.

case 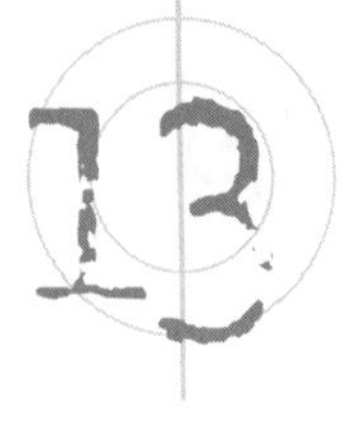

Dilated Cardiomyopathy

Differential

Amyloidosis
Aortic stenosis
Cardiac tamponade
Glycogen storage diseases
Wet beriberi
Thyroid disease

Discussion

Dilated cardiomyopathy may develop in the **peripartum period** (>3 months). Other etiologies include **ischemic heart disease**, **alcoholism** (due to thiamine deficiency or direct toxicity), hypothyroidism, Friedreich ataxia, previous **myocarditis** (usually due to **Coxsackie B**), myotonic dystrophy, chronic hypocalcemia or hypophosphatemia, **sarcoidosis**, and drug toxicities (e.g., **adriamycin**, cyclophosphamide, **tricyclic antidepressants**, **lithium**, and cobalt).

Treatment

Treat cardiac failure with salt restriction, diuretics, vasodilators such as hydralazine (in pregnant patients) or ACE inhibitors (in nonpregnant patients), and digoxin; chronic **anticoagulation**; nutritional supplementation; consider cardiac transplant if medical therapy fails.

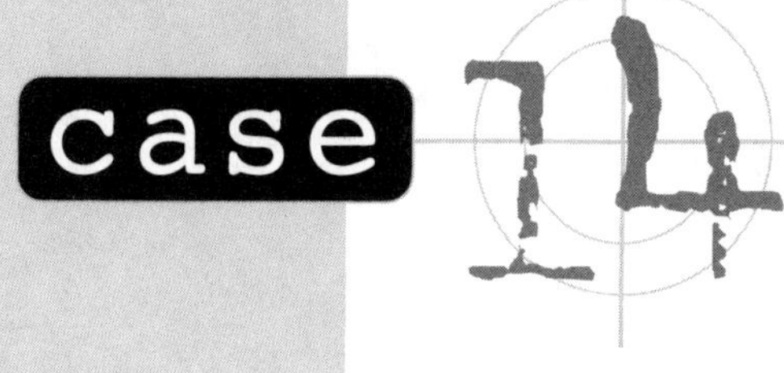

case 14

ID/CC A 23-year-old woman is seen with complaints of **excessive breathlessness, palpitations, fatigue, blood-streaked sputum** (MILD HEMOPTYSIS), **and swelling of the feet** (EDEMA).

HPI She was diagnosed with **ventricular septal defect** (VSD) at birth, but her parents had refused surgery.

PE VS: HR, BP normal; mild tachypnea; no fever. PE: **central cyanosis;** clubbing; predominantly loud P2 (due to pulmonary hypertension); **mid-diastolic murmur** (GRAHAM STEELL MURMUR OF PULMONARY REGURGITATION) **in pulmonary area that increased with inspiration** (CARVALLO SIGN, INDICATING RIGHT-SIDED MURMUR).

Labs ABGs: hypercapnia, hypoxia, and partly compensated respiratory acidosis. CBC: **polycythemia.** ECG: **right ventricular hypertrophy** with right-axis deviation. Cardiac catheterization reveals right-to-left shunt, **pulmonary arterial hypertension.**

Imaging Echo (with Doppler): **VSD with right-to-left systolic shunt;** right ventricular enlargement and hypertrophy. CXR: pulmonary oligemia ("peripheral pruning").

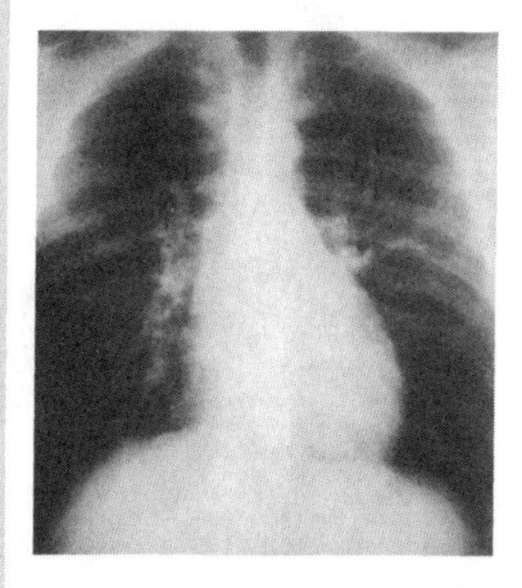

Figure 14-1. The heart is enlarged. There is evidence of increased pulmonary blood flow, and the pulmonary arteries are dilated.

case 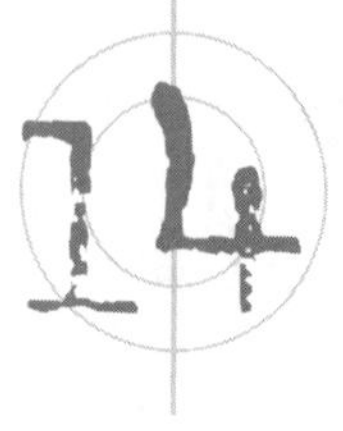

Eisenmenger Complex

Differential

Primary pulmonary hypertension
Tetralogy of Fallot
Restrictive cardiomyopathy

Discussion

The term "Eisenmenger syndrome" applies to those defects in which **pulmonary vascular disease causes right-to-left shunt of blood;** Eisenmenger complex is right-to-left shunt due to a large VSD. The risk of infective endocarditis is high; therefore, antimicrobial prophylaxis is mandatory. Pregnancy is contraindicated owing to a high maternal mortality rate.

Treatment

Heart-lung transplantation; surgical correction of a VSD is ideally performed before irreversible pulmonary vascular changes set in.

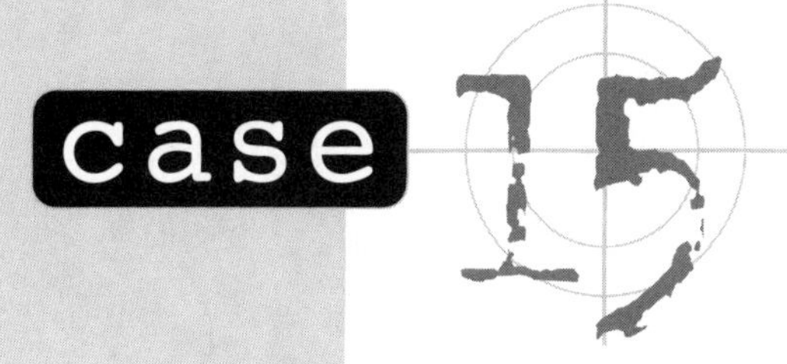

ID/CC A 20-year-old college student is brought back from a summer camp in the mountains after developing **severe shortness of breath** (DYSPNEA), cough with **blood-tinged sputum** (HEMOPTYSIS), and wheezing.

HPI The group had **ascended to a height** of **8,000 feet** and had engaged in **strenuous physical activities.** The patient subsequently developed dyspnea and cough that worsened during the night, leading to **marked respiratory distress and a shocklike state.**

PE VS: tachycardia; tachypnea; hypotension. PE: **central cyanosis;** pale and cold extremities; marked **respiratory distress; widespread rales and rhonchi** over both lung fields.

Labs CBC: **elevated hematocrit and hemoglobin;** mildly increased WBC. ABGs: markedly **decreased arterial** Po_2 (hypoxia); **low** Pco_2**. Increased pH** (respiratory alkalosis). ECG: sinus tachycardia.

Imaging CXR (PA view): **noncardiogenic pulmonary edema** and prominent main pulmonary artery.

Micro Pathology Extensive pulmonary edema; protein-rich exudate with alveolar hemorrhages and **alveolar hyaline membranes.**

case 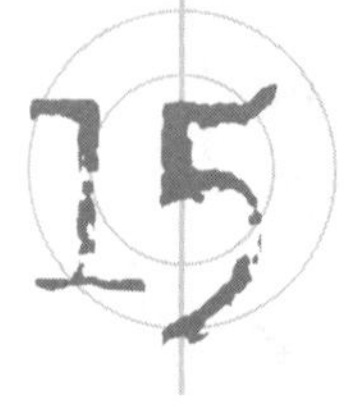

High-Altitude Sickness

Differential

Pulmonary embolism
Bacterial pneumonia
Asthma
Goodpasture syndrome
Viral hemorrhagic syndromes

Discussion

High-altitude pulmonary edema is primarily a disorder of the pulmonary circulation **induced by sustained alveolar hypoxia.** The initiating event is an abnormal degree of **hypoxia-induced pulmonary arteriolar (precapillary) constriction** (hypoxia causes dilatation of systemic blood vessels) that elevates pulmonary arterial pressure. The imbalance of **increased blood flow** and pressure allows fluid to leave the pulmonary vasculature, resulting in **edema.**

Treatment

Prompt descent, hyperbaric oxygen inhalation, sublingual nifedipine (after checking blood pressure), inhaled nitric oxide, and placement in **portable hyperbaric chamber** while being transported; hospital management consists of **continuous high-flow oxygen, dexamethasone for CNS symptoms, and acetazolamide.**

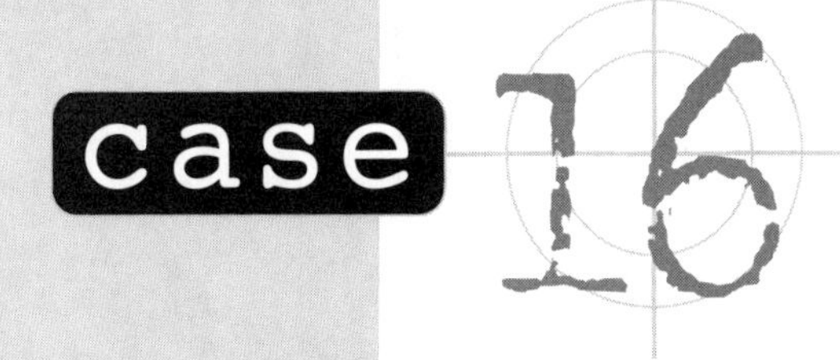

ID/CC	A 21-year-old white mane presents with anginal chest pain, **dyspnea on exertion**, and an episode of **syncope while playing basketball.**
PE	VS: pulse bisferious (DOUBLE PEAKED). Systolic thrill palpable over left sternal border; **S4; ejection systolic murmur** over left third intercostal space radiating to base and axilla; murmur **increased by exercise and during forced expiration against a closed glottis** (VALSALVA MANEUVER) but **decreased by squatting.**
Labs	ECG: left-axis deviation due to **left ventricular hypertrophy.**
Imaging	CXR, PA: often normal. Echo: **asymmetrical septal hypertrophy and systolic anterior motion of mitral valve;** Doppler may show **mitral regurgitation.** Angio, cardiac: marked **thickening of left ventricular septal wall.**
Gross Pathology	**Enlarged heart** with increased weight and **asymmetrical septal hypertrophy.**
Micro Pathology	**Myocyte disarray** with increased norepinephrine content.

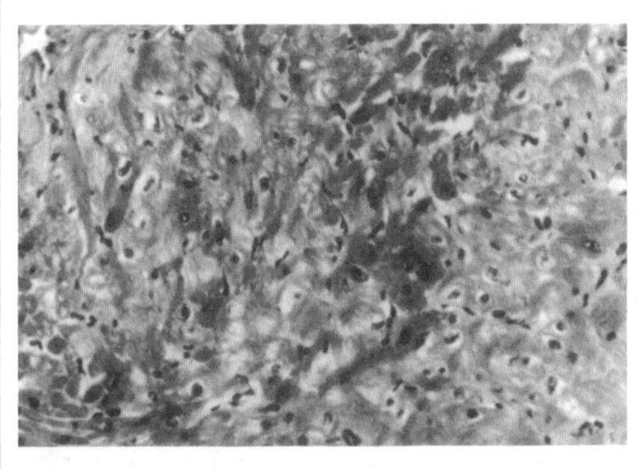

Figure 16-1. Disarray of cardiac fibers.

case 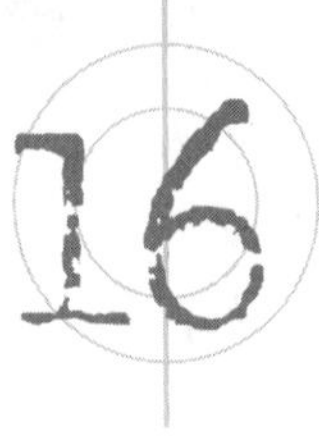

Hypertrophic Cardiomyopathy

Differential

Aortic stenosis
Restrictive cardiomyopathy
Glycogen storage diseases
Fabry disease

Discussion

Also known as **idiopathic hypertrophic subaortic stenosis (IHSS).** An **autosomal dominant** pattern of disease is noted in 50% of cases; ventricular outflow tract obstruction by hypertrophy produces symptoms. The presenting symptom in **athletes** might be **sudden death** secondary to lethal cardiac arrhythmias.

Treatment

Negative inotropic agents (e.g., **beta-blockers,** calcium channel blockers) to decrease stiffness of left ventricle and prevent fatal arrhythmias; **avoidance of competitive sports;** surgical myomectomy of interventricular septum in patients with outflow obstruction.

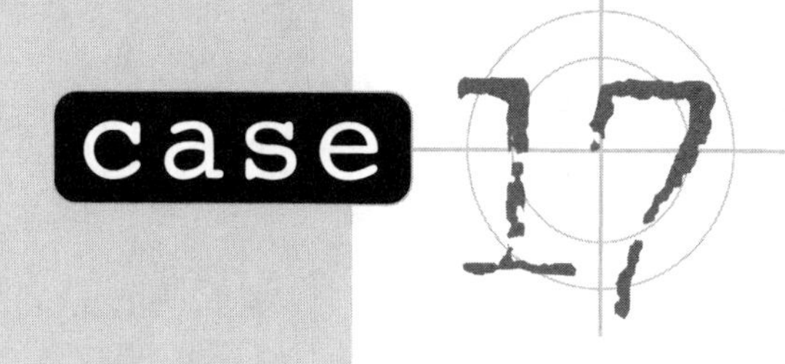

case 17

ID/CC A 28-year-old woman **found on a park bench apparently dead** is brought to the ER in the early hours of the morning.

HPI No discernible pulse was palpated, but a **faint, infrequent respiratory effort was noted;** CPR was begun and continued during her transport to the hospital. The **temperature overnight was near-freezing** with continuous rain.

PE VS: arterial **pulse not palpated;** hypotension; reduced respiratory rate; **severe hypothermia (>28°C).** PE: no respiratory effort; **fixed and dilated pupils;** blotchy areas of erythema on skin; bullae over buttocks; chest exam shows diffuse rales bilaterally; absent bowel sounds; absent deep tendon reflexes.

Labs CBC: increased hematocrit. Hypoglycemia; increased BUN and creatinine. Lytes: decreased bicarbonate; hyperkalemia. ABGs: severe metabolic acidosis. ECG: evidence of **marked bradycardia** with **J (Osborn) waves** (upward waves immediately following the S wave).

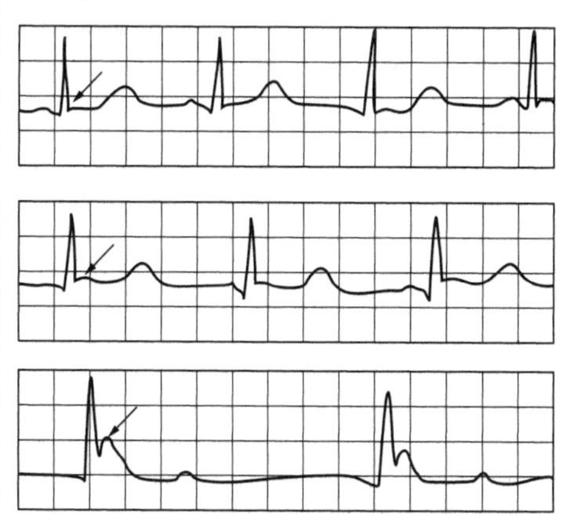

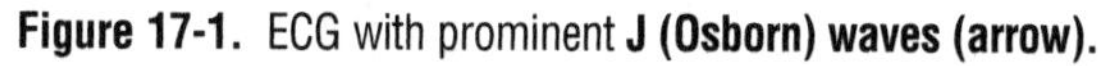

Figure 17-1. ECG with prominent **J (Osborn) waves (arrow).**

Imaging CXR: patchy atelectasis.

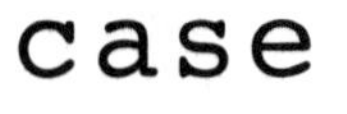
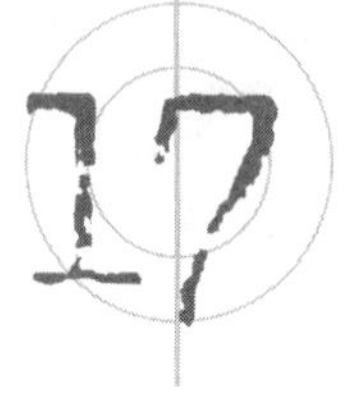

Hypothermia

Differential

Hemorrhagic stroke
Narcotic toxicity
Sedative toxicity
Sepsis
Hypothyroidism

Discussion

Hypothermia is defined as core temperature below 35°C; **severe accidental hypothermia (below 30°C, or 86°F) is associated with marked depression in cerebral blood flow and cerebral oxygen requirement, reduced cardiac output, and decreased arterial pressure.** Victims can **appear to be lifeless** as a result of marked depression of brain function. Peripheral pulses may be difficult to detect because of bradycardia and vasoconstriction. Complications of systemic hypothermia may include ventricular fibrillation, pancreatitis, renal failure, and coagulopathy.

Treatment

Intubation and ventilation as necessary; cardiac massage for arrest; warm the patient through use of a combination of heated blankets, heat packs, warm gastric lavage, warm-water immersion, and high-flow oxygen; monitor cardiac rhythm for arrhythmias.

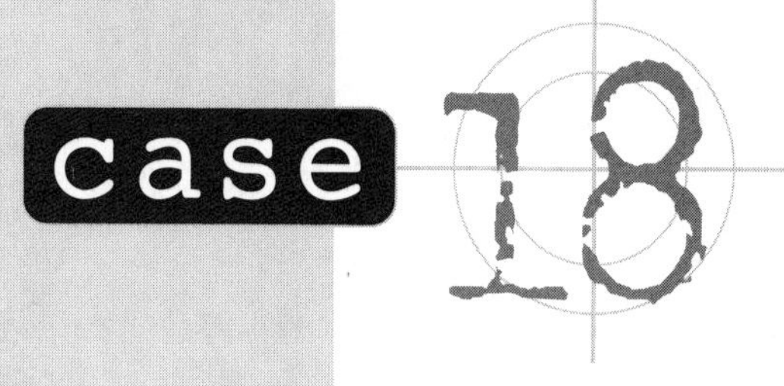

ID/CC A 42-year-old black man presents with **chest pain, headache, altered mental status, and confusion.**

HPI He is known to have **labile essential hypertension.** He has no history of fever.

PE VS: **severe diastolic hypertension** (BP 230/150). PE: **disoriented and confused; bilateral papilledema;** no focal neurologic deficits; remainder of exam normal.

Labs CBC: microangiopathic hemolytic anemia. UA: **hematuria** and **proteinuria. Increased BUN and serum creatinine.** ECG: **left ventricular hypertrophy.**

Imaging CT/US, abdomen: bilateral **small and scarred kidneys.**

Gross Pathology Kidney surface appears "**flea-bitten**" (due to rupture of cortical arterioles and glomerular capillaries).

Micro Pathology Renal biopsy (not routinely indicated) shows **hyperplastic arteriolosclerosis** ("ONION SKINNING") of interlobular arteries with **fibrinoid necrosis** and thrombi in arterioles and small arteries; **necrotizing glomerulitis** with neutrophil infiltration also seen.

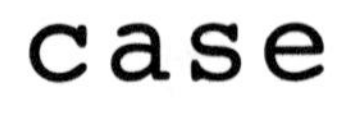
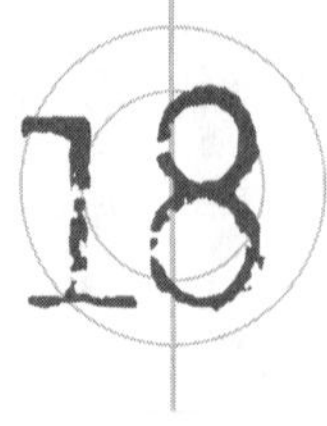

Malignant Hypertension

Differential

Acute coronary syndrome
Aortic dissection
Tension headache
Encephalitis
Pheochromocytoma

Discussion

End-organ damage caused by malignant hypertension includes hemorrhagic and lacunar strokes, encephalopathy, fundal hemorrhages, papilledema, myocardial ischemia/infarction, left ventricular hypertrophy, congestive heart failure, acute renal failure, nephrosclerosis, aortic dissection, and necrotizing vasculitis.

Treatment

Emergent control of hypertension with IV nitroprusside, labetalol, or metoprolol followed by aggressive blood pressure control with oral medications.

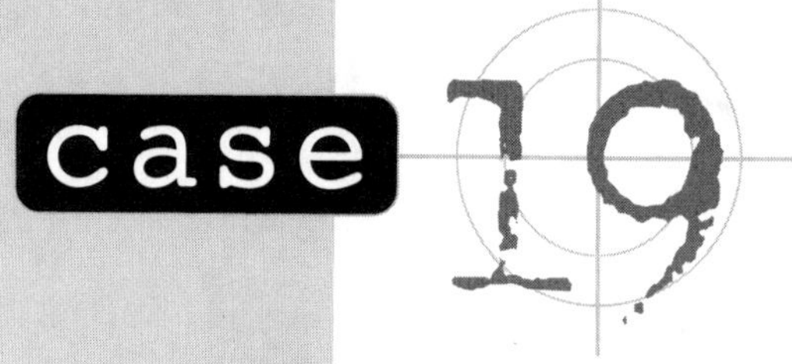

ID/CC The case of a 50-year-old man who died of bleeding complications is discussed at an autopsy meeting owing to **peculiar vegetations seen on his mitral valve.**

HPI He underwent surgery for **adenocarcinoma of the stomach.** Shortly before his death he was diagnosed as having **disseminated intravascular coagulation (DIC)**; he subsequently died of bleeding complications.

Gross Pathology **Small** (1- to 5-mm) **friable, sterile vegetations** loosely adherent to **mitral valve leaflets along lines of closure.**

Micro Pathology Vegetations found to be **sterile fibrin and platelet thrombi** loosely attached **without evidence of inflammation** (bland) or valve damage.

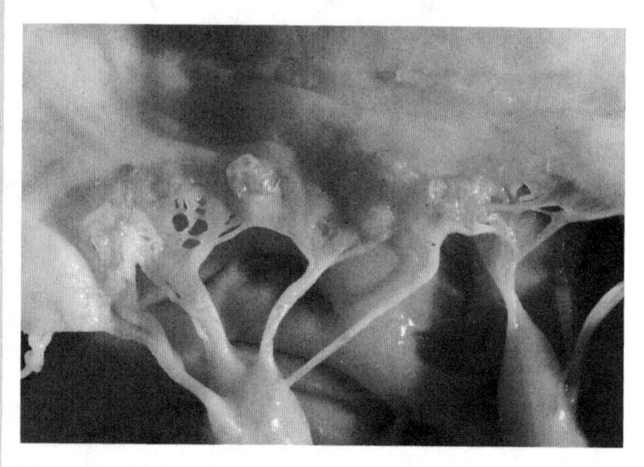

Figure 19-1. Sterile platelet-fibrin vegetations seen on structurally normal valves.

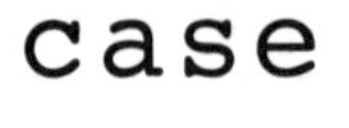

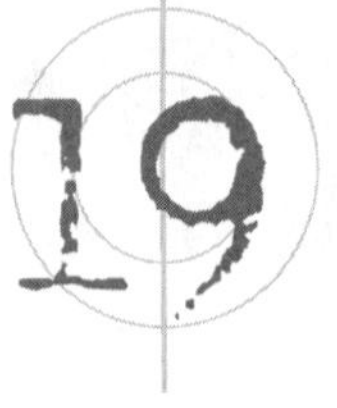

Marantic Endocarditis

Differential

Subacute bacterial endocarditis
Libman–Sacks endocarditis
Rheumatic heart disease
Acute bacterial endocarditis
Carcinoid heart disease

Discussion

Nonbacterial thrombotic endocarditis characteristically occurs in settings of **prolonged debilitating diseases** such as cancer (particularly visceral adenocarcinomas), DIC, renal failure, chronic sepsis, or other **hypercoagulable states.** The vegetations may produce emboli and subsequent infarctions in the heart, kidneys, brain, mesentery, or extremities.

Treatment

Anticoagulation with warfarin in living patients.

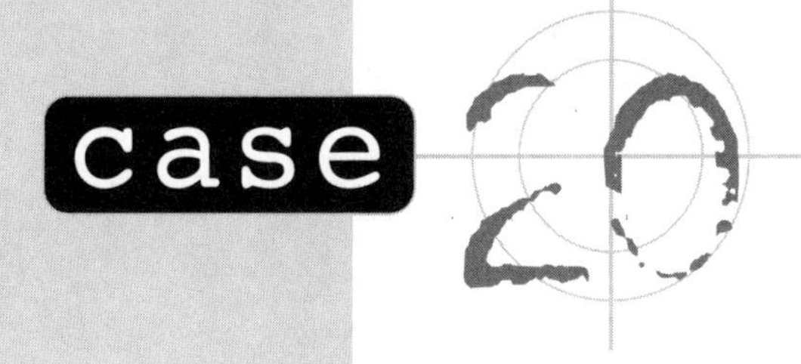

case 20

ID/CC A 17-year-old white girl with **Marfan syndrome** complains of increasing palpitations, dizziness, and what she describes as "panic attacks."

HPI She denies having had any previous history of rheumatic fever.

PE VS: Stable. PE: **Mid-to-late systolic click** with a late systolic murmur.

Labs ECG: left-axis deviation; left atrial and left ventricular hypertrophy.

Imaging CXR/Echo: enlargement of left atrium and ventricle. Displacement of the mitral leaflets 2 mm beyond the mitral annulus.

Gross Pathology Redundant deformed mitral valve leaflets billowing into the left atrial cavity.

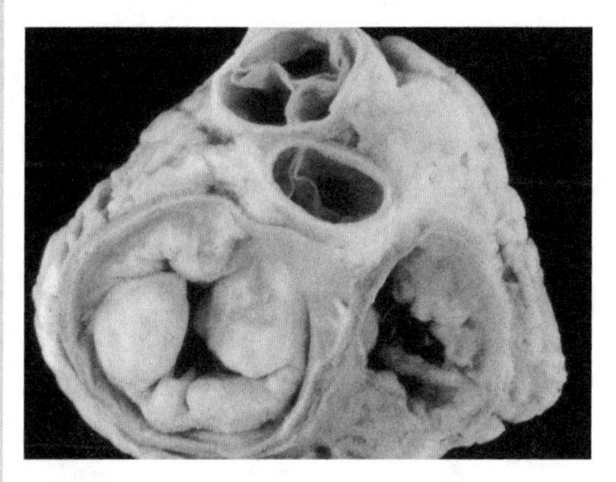

Figure 20-1. Deformed leaflets billowing into left atrium.

Micro Pathology Myxomatous infiltration of the usually dense collagenous valvular and subvalvular tissues.

case

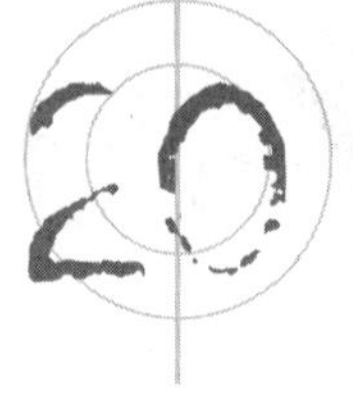

Mitral Insufficiency

Differential

Mitral regurgitation
Connective tissue disease
Mitral stenosis
Pulmonic regurgitation

Discussion

Mitral valve prolapse is the **most common valvular disorder** affecting 2% to 5% of adults. Most are diagnosed on routine physical exam. There is an increased predisposition in patients with connective tissue diseases, including Marfan syndrome, Ehlers–Danlos syndrome, and adult polycystic kidney disease.

Treatment

Oral arteriolar vasodilators (e.g., ACE inhibitors, hydralazine) to improve forward cardiac output; surgical repair or prosthetic replacement; antibiotic prophylaxis with penicillin prior to surgical or dental procedures.

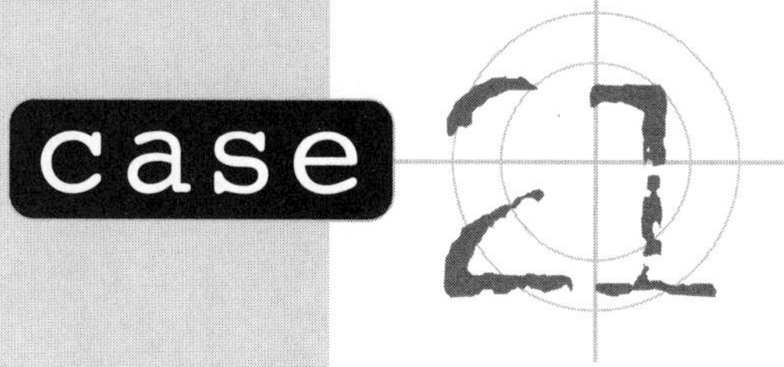

ID/CC A 34-year-old white woman in her 27th week of pregnancy is admitted to the hospital with **dyspnea** and **orthopnea.**

HPI The patient denies any prior cardiovascular disease, but a careful history reveals that she suffered from **streptococcal pharyngitis** and **rheumatic heart disease** as a child.

PE Malar flush; elevated JVP (due to venous congestion); left parasternal heave; loud S1; **opening snap;** rumbling, low-pitched **mid-diastolic murmur** at **apex** heard best in left lateral position.

Labs ECG: **left atrial hypertrophy** and/or **atrial fibrillation.**

Imaging CXR: double silhouette due to enlarged left atrium; Kerley B lines (due to interstitial edema). Echo: **leaflet thickening** with **fusion of the commissures.**

Gross Pathology Thickening and fusion of the mitral valve leaflets with significant narrowing of the orifice, "**fish mouth deformity.**"

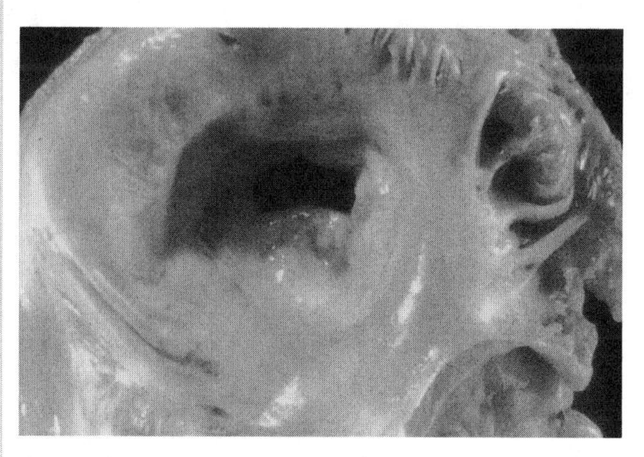

Figure 21-1. Fish mouth deformity.

case 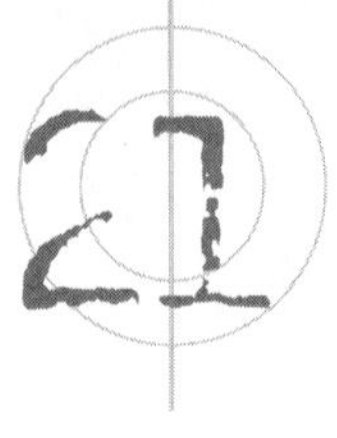

Mitral Stenosis

Differential

Mitral regurgitation

Mitral valve prolapse

Hypertrophic obstructive cardiomyopathy

Myocardial infarction

Discussion

The most common cause of mitral stenosis is rheumatic heart disease. The main changes to the valve include leaflet thickening, fusion of the commissures, and shortening, thickening, and fusion of the cordae tendineae.

Treatment

Diuretics to relieve pulmonary congestion; treatment of concomitant atrial fibrillation with ventricular rate control (using digoxin) and anticoagulation; valvuloplasty or prosthetic valve replacement; antibiotic prophylaxis against infective endocarditis prior to surgical or dental procedures.

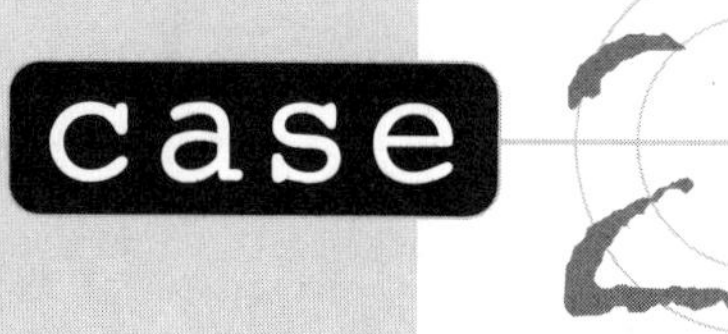

case 22

ID/CC An 18-year-old white **boy** complains of gradually progressing **shortness of breath** and **ankle swelling.**

HPI His symptoms started following a **URI.** He also complains of **excessive fatigue and frequent chest pain.**

PE VS: tachycardia; hypotension; no fever. PE: **elevated JVP;** pitting pedal edema; fine inspiratory rales at both lung bases; mild tender hepatomegaly; splenomegaly; **right-sided S3;** murmurs of mitral regurgitation.

Labs ASO titers not raised. CBC: lymphocytosis. Elevated ESR. ECG: **first-degree AV block with nonspecific ST-T** changes. Increased titers of serum antibodies to Coxsackie virus; **elevated cardiac enzymes.**

Imaging CXR: cardiomegaly and pulmonary edema.

Gross Pathology Flabby, dilated heart with foci of myocardial petechial hemorrhages.

Micro Pathology Endomyocardial biopsy reveals **diffuse infiltration by mononuclear cells, predominantly lymphocytes;** interstitial edema; focal myofiber necrosis; focal fibrosis.

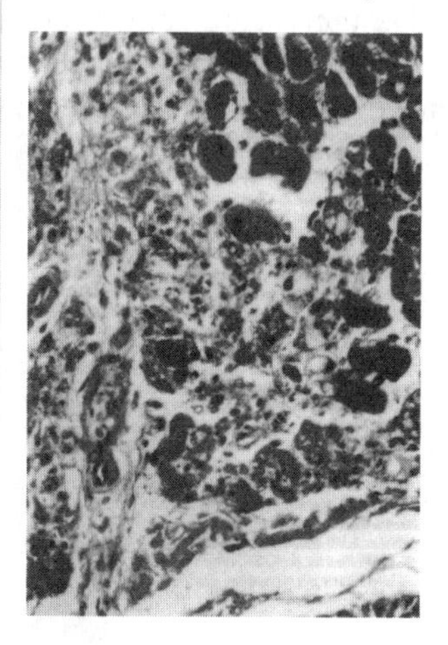

Figure 22-1. Extensive inflammatory infiltrate with myocyte necrosis.

case 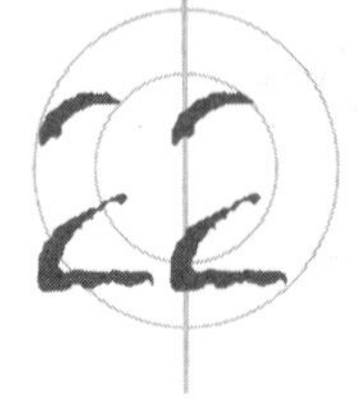

Myocarditis

Differential

Cardiomyopathy
Coronary vasospasm
Myocardial infarction
Cardiac tamponade
Congestive heart failure

Discussion

The etiology of myocarditis is usually **Coxsackie B** or other viruses; less often implicated are bacteria or fungi, rickettsiae (e.g., Rocky Mountain spotted fever), spirochetes (e.g., Lyme disease), *Trypanosoma cruzi* (Chagas disease), hypersensitivity disease (SLE, drug reaction), radiation, and sarcoidosis. Diphtheria toxin also causes myocarditis by inhibiting eukaryotic elongation factor 2 (EF-2), thus inhibiting myocyte protein synthesis. It may also be idiopathic. Young males are primarily affected.

Treatment

Rest; specific antimicrobial therapy when appropriate; control of congestive cardiac failure by diuretics, digitalis, and vasodilators; antiarrhythmics if indicated; cardiac transplant in intractable cases. Although most cases of acute myocarditis may resolve spontaneously, some progress to dilated cardiomyopathy.

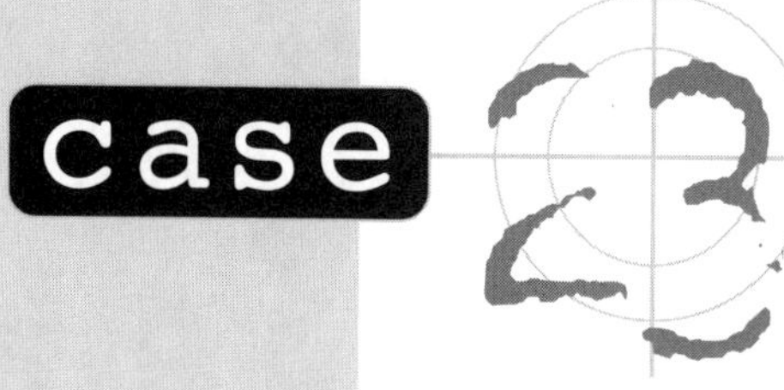

ID/CC A 64-year-old white woman complains of **sudden-onset severe pain** in her left leg with **associated weakness** of the left foot. The pain intensifies when she moves her leg, and she cannot move her toes at all.

HPI She is a **smoker** and has a history of **limited exercise tolerance** due to **pain in her lower extremities** (INTERMITTENT CLAUDICATION).

PE VS: normal. PE: lipid deposition in skin (XANTHELASMAS); popliteal, dorsalis pedis, and posterior tibial **pulses lost** on left side; femoral pulses easily palpable; left leg **cold and mottled; anesthesia** over lower left leg.

Labs CBC: leukocytosis.

Imaging US, Doppler: obstruction of left common iliac. Angio: confirmatory; assess runoff and collaterals prior to surgery.

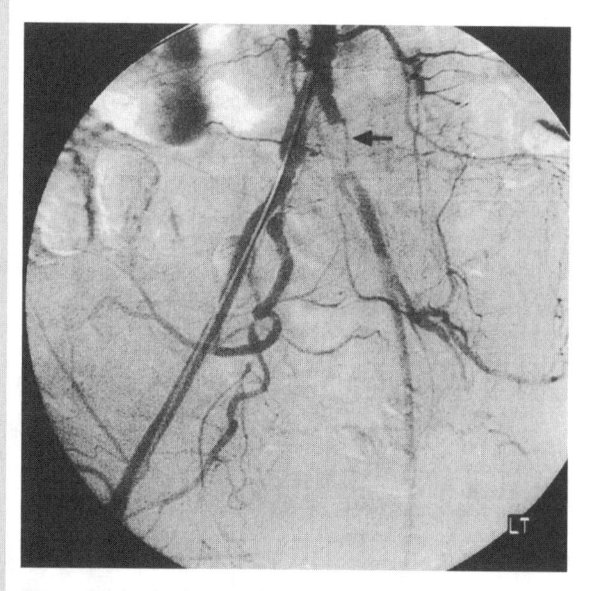

Figure 23-1. Angiogram demonstrating occlusion of the left common iliac.

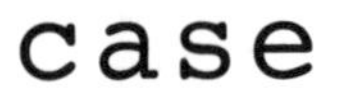
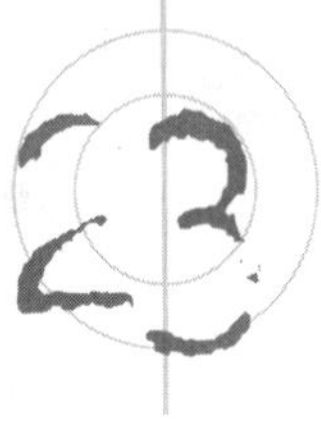

Peripheral Arterial Embolism

Differential

Pseudoclaudication
Buerger disease
Popliteal artery entrapment
Diabetic neuropathy

Discussion

Arterial embolism may have various causes, such as **atrial fibrillation, myocardial infarction, prosthetic heart valves,** endocarditis, cancer, dilated cardiomyopathy, **paradoxical embolism** from the venous system, or a dislodged mural thrombus from an **abdominal aortic aneurysm** or an atheromatous plaque. The earlier the intervention, the higher the likelihood that the limb may be salvaged. Clinically characterized by the **five P's: pain, pallor, paralysis, paresthesia, and pulselessness.**

Treatment

Thrombolysis; consider embolectomy.

Breakout Point

The 5 P's of peripheral arterial occlusion
- Paresthesis
- Pain
- Pallor
- Pulselessness
- Paralysis

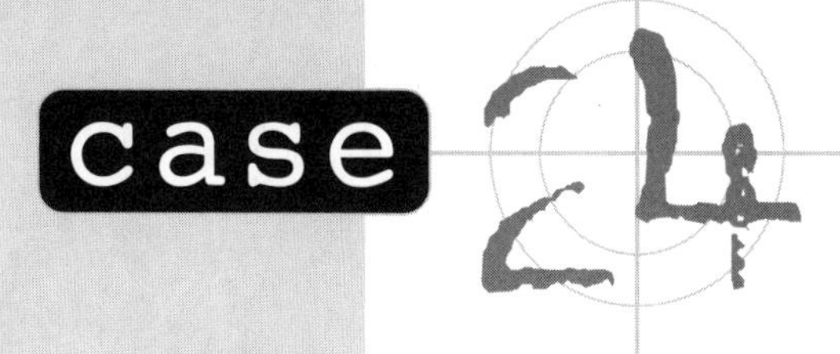

ID/CC A 25-year-old woman is brought to the ER after having sustained a stab wound on her left thigh following a drunken brawl.

HPI A tourniquet was tied above the site, which the attendants said was **spurting blood like "a tap run open."**

PE VS: **hypotension;** weak, fast pulse. PE: anxious and confused; **cool skin with reduced capillary filling;** very **low central venous pressure;** releasing tourniquet confirmed femoral artery puncture.

Labs CBC: mildly decreased hematocrit. BUN and creatinine normal. Lytes: normal.

Imaging Arteriogram shows abrupt termination of dye propagation in the common femoral artery.

case 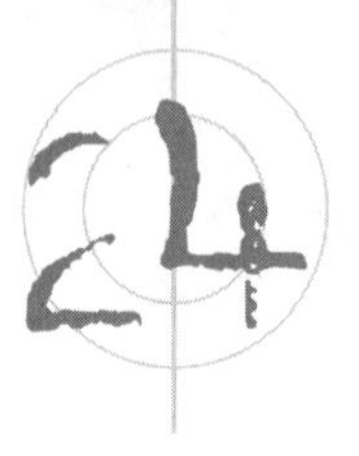

Shock—Hypovolemic

Differential

Ectopic pregnancy
Abdominal aortic aneurysm
Pelvic fracture
Thoracic aneurysm
Gastrointestinal bleed

Discussion

The clinical conditions that cause hypovolemic shock include **acute and subacute hemorrhage and dehydration;** fluid loss into an extravascular compartment can significantly reduce intravascular volume and result in nonhemorrhagic hypovolemic shock. Acute pancreatitis, loss of the enteral integument (from conditions such as burns and surgical wounds), or occlusive or dynamic ileus can all induce oligemic hypotension as a result of extravasation of fluids into the extracellular compartment. Other forms of water and solute loss, such as diarrhea, hyperglycemia (leading to glucosuria), diabetes insipidus, salt-wasting nephritis, protracted vomiting, adrenocortical failure, acute peritonitis, and overzealous use of diuretics, can also lead to decreased intravascular volume and hypovolemic shock. Patients with prolonged tissue hypoperfusion may progress to metabolic acidosis.

Treatment

Arrest of femoral artery hemorrhage with vascular repair; intensive IV fluid therapy using normal saline and cross-matched blood transfusions; supplemental oxygen; close monitoring of pulse rate, blood pressure, urine output, and central venous pressure.

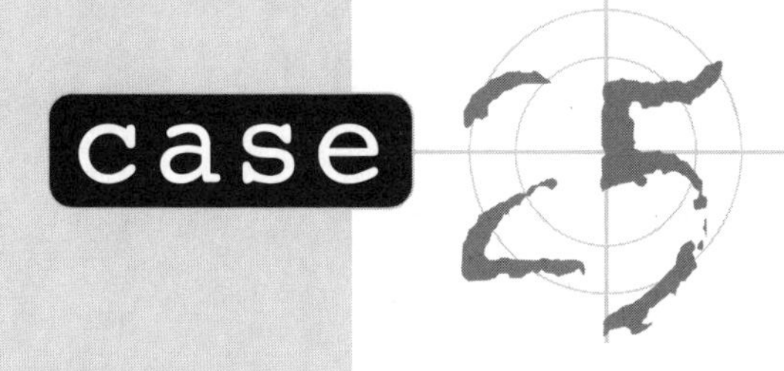

ID/CC A 29-year-old-man is referred to a cardiology clinic for evaluation for a permanent pacemaker.

HPI The patient is asymptomatic and denies dizziness, syncope, chest pain, or shortness of breath. He was incidentally noted to have slow heart rate. He is a **marathon runner** and works as a ranger in a national park, often at elevations above 8,000 feet.

PE VS: no fever, **mild hypotension (BP 90/50) without orthostasis; slow heart rate (HR 40).** PE: thin and athletic-looking; normal JVP; S1 and S2 normally auscultated without any murmurs, gallops, and/or rubs; no lower extremity edema.

Labs CBC/Lytes: normal. ECG: marked reduction in heart rate with a ventricular rate of **40 beats/minute.**

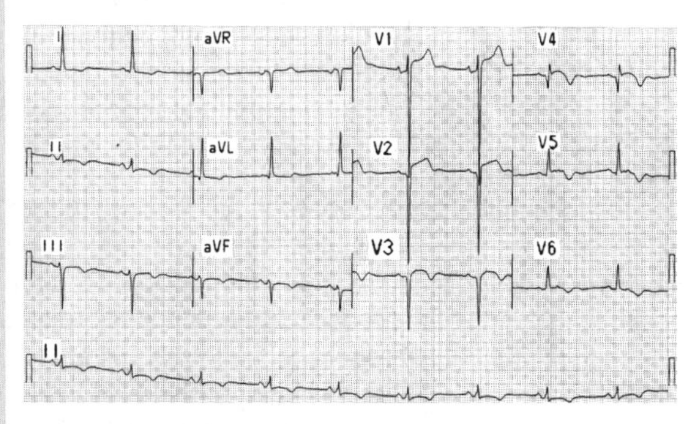

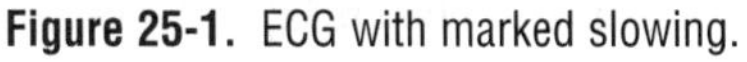
Figure 25-1. ECG with marked slowing.

Imaging XR, chest: normal.

case

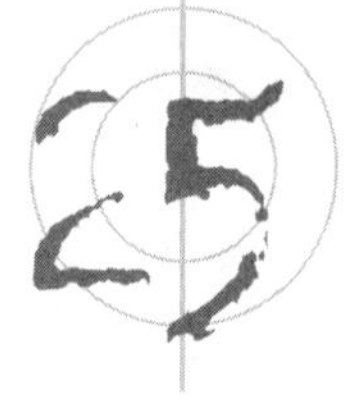

Sinus Bradycardia

Differential

Hypoglycemia
Hypothermia
Hypothyroidism
Digitalis toxicity
Beta-blocker toxicity

Discussion

Sinus bradycardia is defined as a sinus rhythm with a resting heart rate of less than **60 beats/minute.** Physiologic causes of sinus bradycardia include **increased vagal tone** seen in athletes and incidental findings in **young** or **sleeping** patients. Pathologic causes include **inferior wall myocardial infarction, toxic or environmental exposure (dimethyl sulfoxide, toluene), electrolyte disorders, infection, sleep apnea, drug effects (digitalis glycosides, beta-blockers, amiodarone, calcium channel blockers), hypoglycemia, hypothyroidism,** and **increased intracranial pressure.** The most common cause of symptomatic sinus bradycardia is **sick sinus syndrome.**

Treatment

In emergent situations, treat **symptomatic sinus bradycardia** with IV access, supplemental oxygen, and cardiac monitoring. IV atropine may be used in symptomatic patients. Correct all underlying electrolyte and acid–base disorders or hypoxia. Address cause of bradycardia. This patient has a **physiologic sinus bradycardia,** and thus no treatment is indicated.

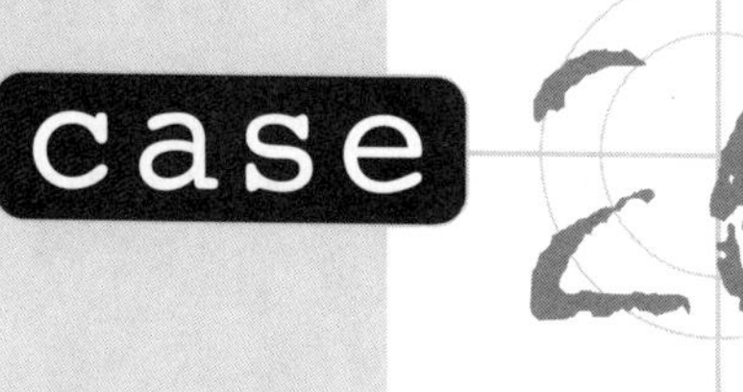

case 26

ID/CC A 50-year-old man presents with complaints of **palpitations** and **chest pain.**

HPI The pain increases with physical activity and is relieved by rest. He has **multiple sexual partners.**

PE VS: high-volume, **collapsing pulse** (WATER-HAMMER PULSE); **wide pulse pressure.** PE: pistol shots heard over brachial artery; to-and-fro murmur heard over femoral artery (DUROZIEZ MURMUR); cardiomegaly; loud aortic component of S2; grade III **early diastolic murmur** heard radiating down right sternal edge (murmur of aortic incompetence); mid-diastolic murmur heard at apex (AUSTIN FLINT MURMUR).

Labs ECG: **left ventricular hypertrophy** with strain pattern. **VDRL and FTA-ABS positive.**

Imaging CXR: **"tree bark" calcification** of ascending aorta and arch of aorta; **mediastinal widening and cardiomegaly.** Echo: **aortic incompetence.**

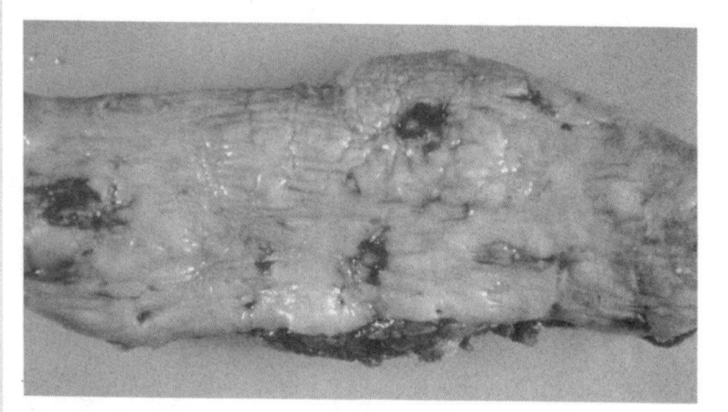

Figure 26-1. The thoracic aorta is dilated, and its inner surface shows the typical "tree bark" appearance.

Gross Pathology Gross cardiac hypertrophy (cor bovinum); **aortic aneurysm** involving the **arch** and the **ascending aorta** and extending into the aortic valve.

Micro Pathology **Obliterative endarteritis** of vasa vasorum.

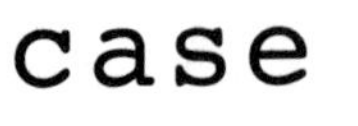
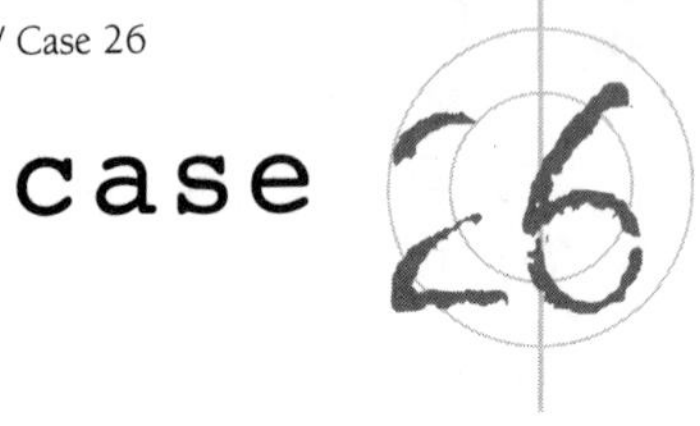

Syphilis—Tertiary (Aortitis)

Differential

Mycotic aneurysm
Aortic dissection
Giant cell arteritis
Cystic medial necrosis

Discussion

Aortitis occurs in the **tertiary stage of syphilis**, often arising many decades after the primary infection. Weakening of the aortic wall causes dilatation of the aortic root as well as aortic incompetence and aneurysms. Intimal fibrosis causes narrowing of the openings of the coronary arteries (ostial stenosis), resulting in myocardial ischemia.

Treatment

Penicillin; surgical excision and repair.

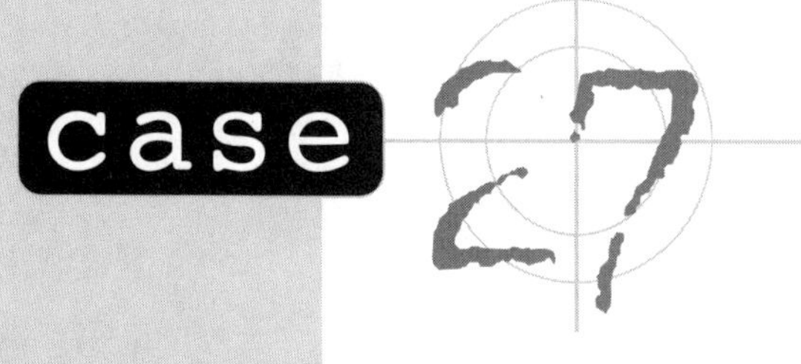

case 27

ID/CC A **35-year-old man** complains of severe, **cramping pains in his calves that prevent him from walking** (INTERMITTENT CLAUDICATION).

HPI The patient states that the pain comes mainly after playing basketball. More recently it has appeared, accompanied by numbness, following mild exertion and **at rest** (due to progression of disease). He admits to **smoking** up to three packs of cigarettes per day.

PE Painful, cordlike indurations of veins (sequelae of **migratory superficial thrombophlebitis**); **pallor**; cyanosis; coldness; diminished peripheral artery pulsations; **Raynaud phenomenon**; delayed return of hand color following release of temporarily occluded radial artery while exercising hand. **Necrosis of the fingertips of several digits.**

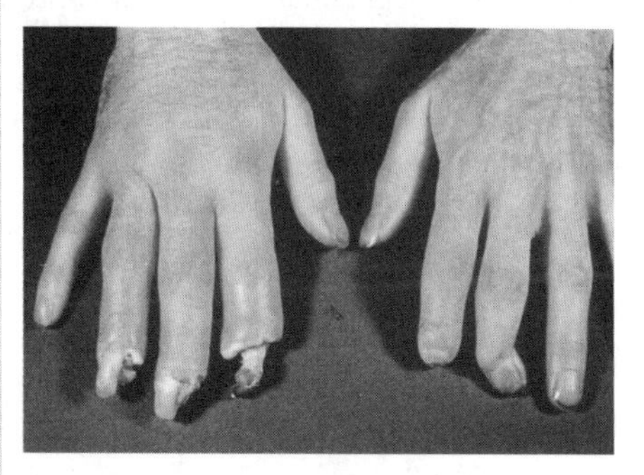

Figure 27-1. Severe involvement of the distal extremities with necrosis of the fingertips.

Imaging Angio, peripheral: **multiple occluded segments** of small and medium-sized arteries in lower leg and arms.

Gross Pathology Arterial segmental thrombosis; **no atherosclerosis**; secondary **gangrene** of leg if severe.

Micro Pathology Segmental vasculitis with round cell infiltration in **all layers** of arterial wall; inflammation; thrombosis; microabscess formation.

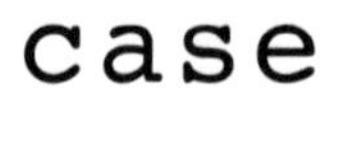

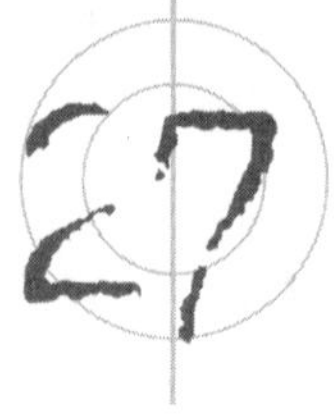

Thromboangiitis Obliterans—Buerger Disease

Differential

Frostbite

Giant cell arteritis

Peripheral arterial occlusive disease

Diabetic neuropathy

Systemic lupus erythematosus

Discussion

Thromboangiitis obliterans tends to affect medium-size and small arteries of the distal extremities. If smoking is not discontinued, multiple finger and toe amputations may be necessary.

Treatment

Cessation of smoking critical; avoidance of exposure to cold and other vasoconstriction-inducing agents; sympathectomy; amputation. Surgical revascularization is usually not possible owing to diffuse and segmental involvement and to the distal nature of the disease.

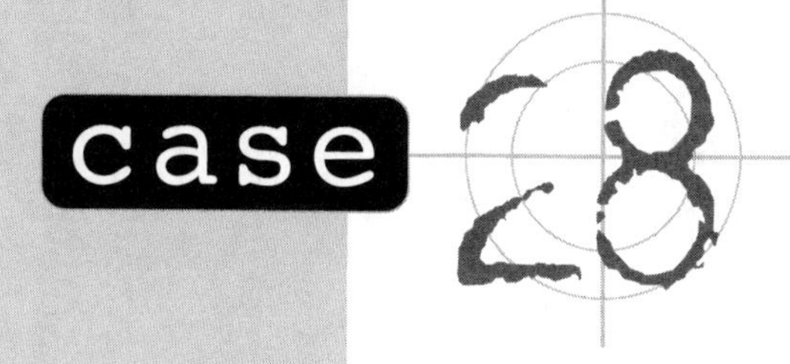

ID/CC A 50-year-old woman who was admitted to the hospital for treatment of staphylococcal endocarditis complains of **severe pain at the site of antibiotic infusion.**

HPI She was receiving **cloxacillin** in addition to penicillin and gentamycin.

PE Markedly **tender, cordlike inflamed area** found at site of infusion.

Gross Pathology Intraluminal venous thrombus adherent to the vessel wall.

Micro Pathology Acute inflammatory cells with endothelial wall damage and intraluminal thrombosis.

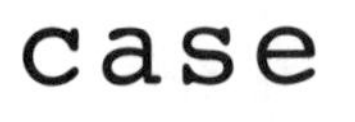
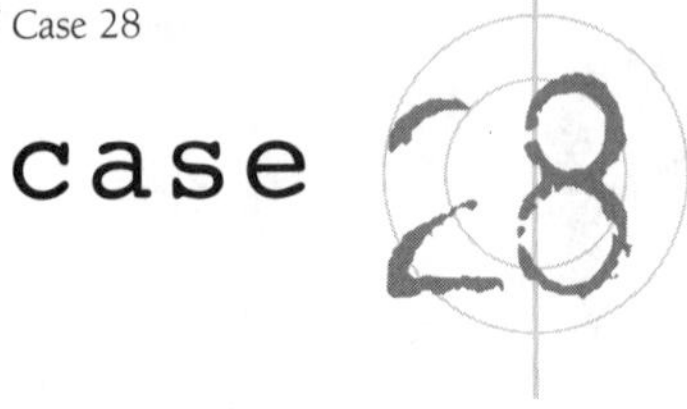

Thrombophlebitis—Superficial

Differential

Cellulitis
Deep vein thrombosis
Chronic venous insufficiency
Lymphedema
Varicosities

Discussion

Superficial thrombophlebitis most commonly occurs in **varicose veins** or in **veins cannulated for an infusion.** Spontaneous thrombophlebitis may occur in conditions such as pregnancy, polycythemia, polyarteritis nodosa, and Buerger disease (thromboangiitis obliterans) and as a sign of visceral cancer (thrombophlebitis migrans—Trousseau sign).

Treatment

Change infusion site frequently; NSAIDs and local heat; support and bed rest.

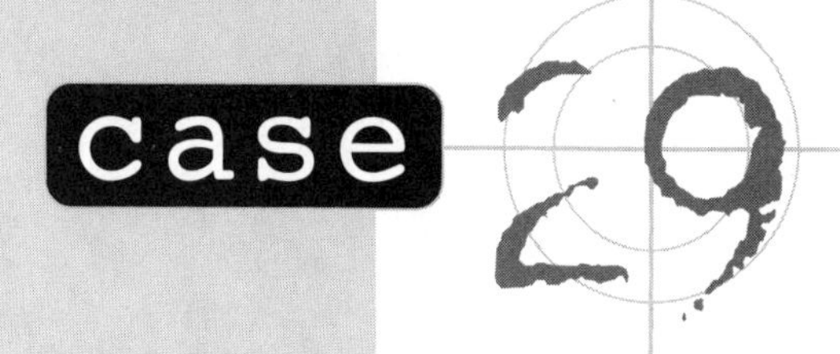

ID/CC A 15-year-old boy is referred to a cardiologist by a primary care physician for an evaluation of **recurrent dizzy spells.**

HPI During his episodes he feels **intense anxiety with palpitations and breathlessness.** He has no history of chest pain or syncope and is normal in between episodes of dizziness.

PE General and systemic physical exam normal; cardiac exam normal; otologic causes ruled out.

Labs ECG: **short PR interval, wide QRS complex, and a slurred upstroke** ("DELTA WAVE") **of QRS complex; R wave in V1 positive.** Electrophysiologic studies confirm **presence of a bypass tract** and its potential for development of life-threatening arrhythmia.

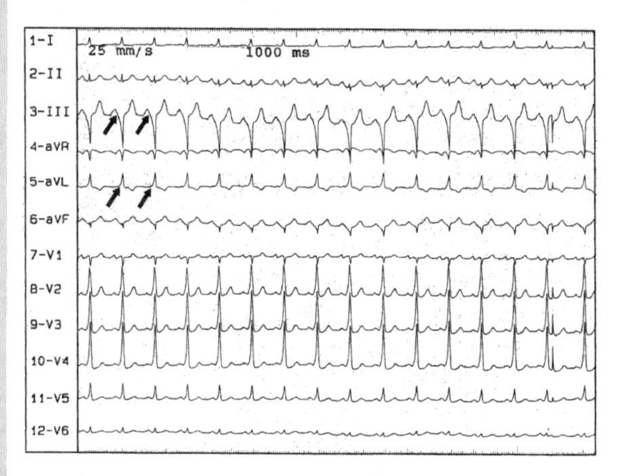

Figure 29-1. The PR interval is short, and there is marked slurring of the onset of the QRS (delta wave: arrow).

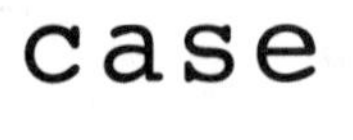
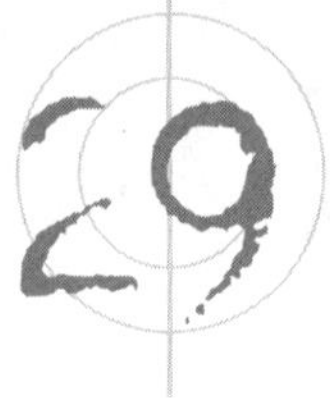

Wolff–Parkinson–White Syndrome

Differential

Nodal re-entry tachycardia
Ebstein abnormality
Syncopy
Atrial fibrillation
Atrial flutter

Discussion

Wolff–Parkinson–White (WPW) syndrome is a term that is applied to patients with both pre-excitation on ECG and paroxysmal tachycardia; in this case, the spells of dizziness could have been either paroxysmal supraventricular tachycardia or atrial fibrillation. In WPW syndrome, an accessory pathway (Kent bundle) exists between the atria and ventricles. An atrial premature contraction or a ventricular premature contraction generally initiates the re-entrant tachycardia, with the accessory tract usually conducting in a retrograde manner; the danger of atrial fibrillation lies in the fact that the accessory pathway may be capable of conducting very fast atrial rates, leading to a fast ventricular response that may degenerate into ventricular arrhythmias.

Treatment

Catheter radiofrequency ablation of the accessory tract is the treatment of choice. Because digitalis reduces the refractory period of the accessory tract, it should be avoided.

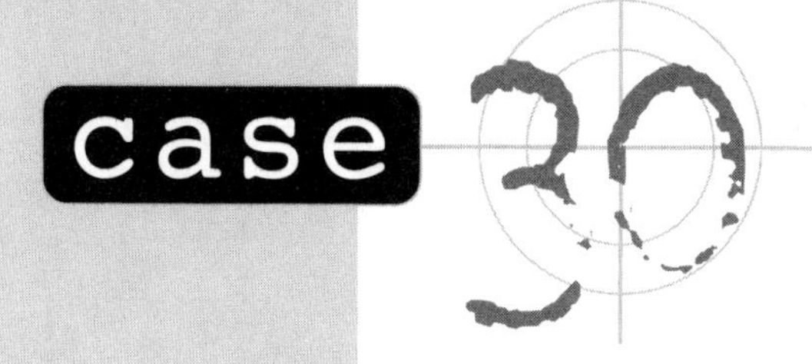

ID/CC A **60-year-old white farmer** presents with skin lesions on his **forehead, above his upper lip, and on the dorsum of his hands.**

HPI He does not smoke, drink alcohol, or chew tobacco.

PE Round or irregularly shaped lesions; tan plaques with adherent **scaly or rough surface** on forehead, skin over upper lip, forearms, and dorsum of hands; lesions range in size from several millimeters to 1 cm or more.

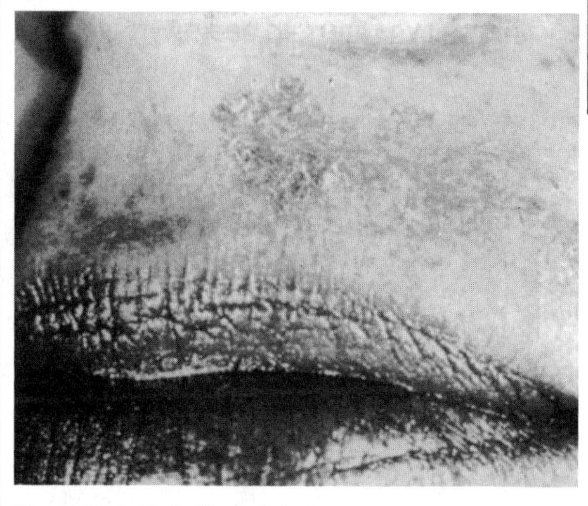

Figure 30-1. Typically scaly lesions on sun-exposed upper lip.

Micro Pathology Epidermis thickened with basal cell hyperplasia; atypical cells tend to invade most superficial portion of the dermis, which shows thickening and fibrosis (ELASTOSIS).

case 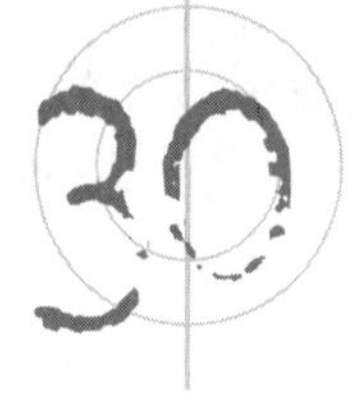

Actinic Keratosis

Differential

Basal cell carcinoma
Discoid lupus
Seborrheic keratosis
Squamous cell carcinoma

Discussion

Also known as senile or **solar keratosis**, actinic keratosis is the most common **precancerous dermatosis** and may progress to **squamous cell carcinoma.** It occurs most commonly in **fair-skinned** individuals and in older persons. Signs that actinic keratosis has become malignant are elevation, ulceration or inflammation, and recent enlargement (>1 cm). Immunosuppressed patients are at high risk of developing actinic keratosis with **prolonged sun exposure.** Look for multiple lesions and for newly developed lesions; **biopsy all suspicious lesions.**

Treatment

Liquid-nitrogen cryotherapy; topical treatment with fluorouracil; surgical excision; electrodesiccation; minimize sun exposure.

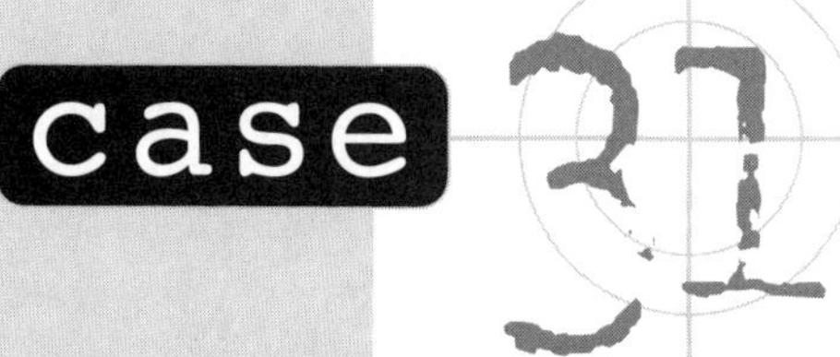

ID/CC A 12-year-old boy presents with severe **itching** and burning at the back of both knees.

HPI He has had similar episodes since the age of 7. His **mother** suffers from **asthma** and his **father** had a **similar skin ailment.**

PE VS: no fever. PE: perioral pallor, increased palmar markings, and **extra fold of skin below the lower eyelid** (DENNIE LINE); **erythematous, vesicular, weeping, rough patchy skin rash** in both popliteal fossae with thickening, crusting, and scaling on the peripheries.

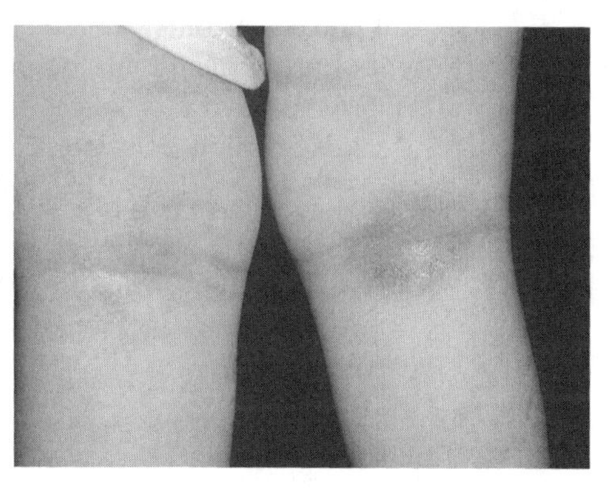

Figure 31-1. Involvement of flexural areas.

Labs CBC: **eosinophilia. High serum IgE levels.**

Micro Pathology Skin biopsy reveals lymphocytic infiltrate with edematous intercellular spaces in the epidermis and prominent intercellular bridges; splayed keratinocytes located primarily in the stratum spinosum.

case 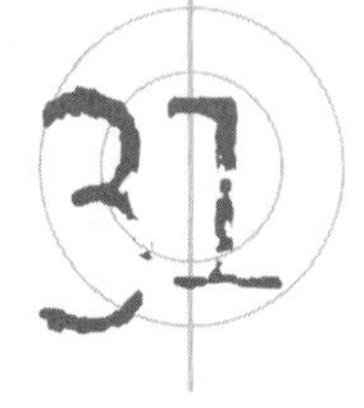

Atopic Dermatitis

Differential

Contact dermatitis
Psoriasis
Scabies
Wiskott–Aldrich syndrome
Drug reaction

Discussion

Clinical criteria for the diagnosis of atopic dermatitis include recurrent episodes of pruritus lasting more than 6 weeks with a personal or family history of atopy and skin lesions typical of eczematous dermatitis.

Treatment

Avoidance of skin irritants; low- or midpotency **topical glucocorticoids;** antihistamines; systemic antibiotics (for secondary infection). Severe exacerbations unresponsive to topical steroids may need systemic steroids or immunosuppressive therapy.

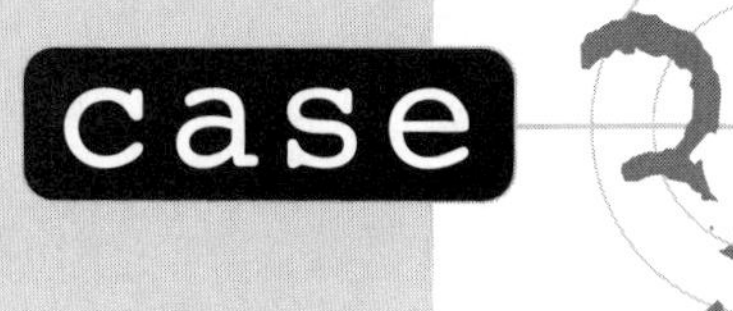

case 32

ID/CC A 68-year-old **red-haired white** man presents with a 3-month history of a progressively **raised, bleeding, ulcerated lesion** in front of his ear that has not responded to various ointments.

HPI He is a **farmer** and has always **worked outdoors**; he occasionally smokes but does not drink.

PE Large, **ill-defined, telangiectatic and ulcerated nodule** ("PEARLY PAPULE") with heaped-up borders located in front of right ear; no regional lymphadenopathy.

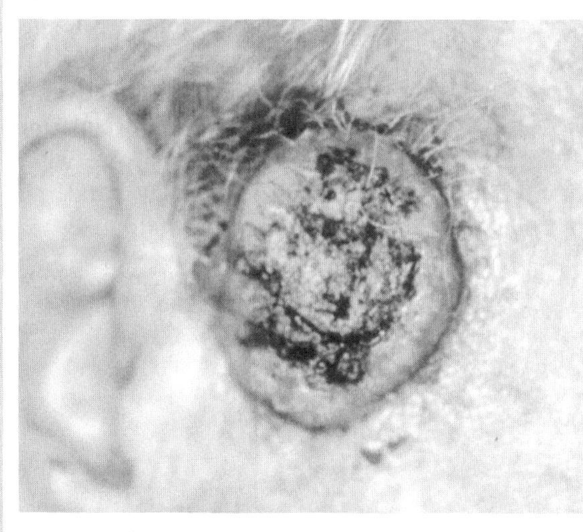

Figure 32-1. Raised, bleeding, ulcerated lesion.

Gross Pathology Generally local but sometimes extensive destruction.

Micro Pathology Biopsy shows basophilic cells with scant cytoplasm as well as palisading basal cells with atypia and increased mitotic index.

case

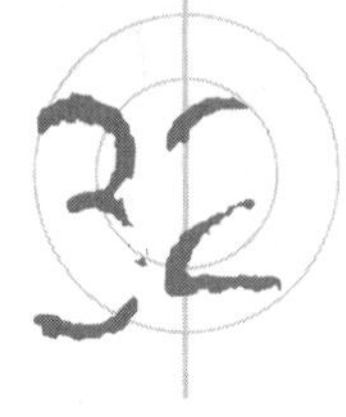

Basal Cell Carcinoma

Differential

Squamous cell carcinoma
Eczema
Molluscum contagiosum
Dermatitis
Angiofibroma

Discussion

Basal cell carcinoma typically occurs in **light-skinned people. The most common skin cancer,** it is seen mainly on **sun-exposed areas** (e.g., face, nose) and is very slow growing. **Metastatic disease is rare** (<0.17%); **chronic, prolonged exposure to sun** is the most important risk factor. Other risk factors include **male gender, advanced age, fair complexion,** and **outdoor occupations.** An increased incidence is seen in people with defective DNA repair mechanisms (e.g., xeroderma pigmentosum) and immunosuppression.

Treatment

Surgical excision with biopsy; cryosurgery; electrodesiccation.

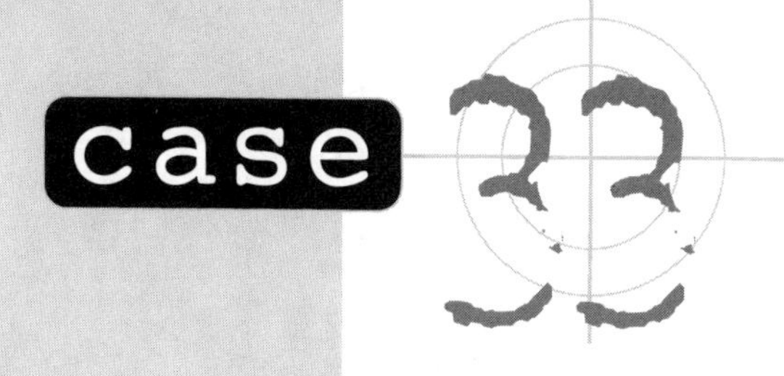

case 33

ID/CC An 8-year-old boy presents with **intense pruritus and fluid-filled blisters** over his arms and legs.

HPI He recently went on a camping trip with his classmates, during which he played the whole day in the bushes around the camping site.

PE Typical **linear streaked vesicles over both arms and legs and back;** weepy and encrusted areas; numerous scratch marks over skin.

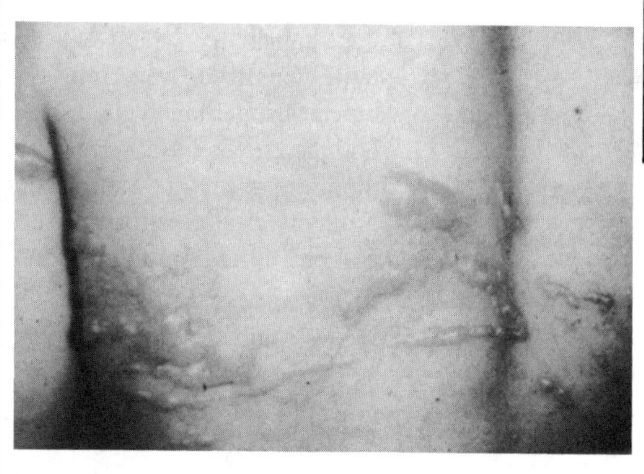

Figure 33-1. Linear streaked vesicles.

Labs Gram stain and culture to rule out secondary infection; KOH preparation negative.

Gross Pathology Skin erythema and edema, with linear streaked vesicles.

Micro Pathology Superficial perivascular **lymphocytic infiltration** around the blood vessels associated with edema of the dermal papillae and mast cell degranulation.

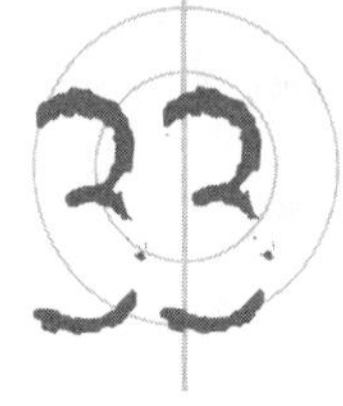

Contact Dermatitis

Differential

Insect bite
Atopic dermatitis
Herpes zoster
Impetigo
Scabies

Discussion

While at the campground the boy probably encountered poison ivy, a plant that produces low-molecular-weight oils (URUSHIOLS) that induce contact hypersensitivity, which is a **cell-mediated, type IV hypersensitivity reaction.** The antigen is presented by the Langerhans cells to the helper lymphocytes. Both cell types travel to regional lymph nodes, where the antigen presentation is increased. Upon antigen challenge, the sensitized T cells infiltrate the dermis and begin the immune response.

Treatment

Systemic and oral steroids.

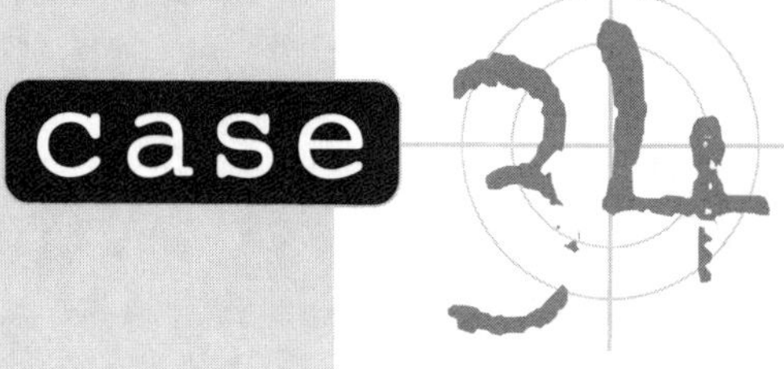

ID/CC A 35-year-old **man** presents with an **intensely pruritic rash** on his **elbows, knees, and back.**

HPI He has **celiac sprue** and observes prescribed dietary precautions (gluten restriction).

PE PE: **bilaterally symmetrical** polymorphic skin lesions in the form of **small, tense vesicles on erythematous skin**; bullae and groups of papules over scapular and sacral areas, knees and elbows, and other **extensor surfaces.**

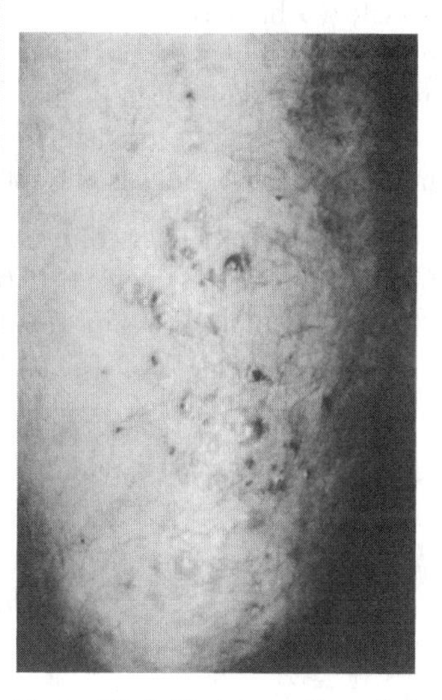

Figure 34-1. Vesicles and multiple crusted (i.e., excoriated) lesions on the elbow.

Labs **HLA-B8/DR-w3** haplotype (particularly prone).

Gross Pathology **Polymorphous erythematous lesions**, including **papules, small vesicles**, and **larger bullae.**

Micro Pathology Skin biopsy reveals characteristic **subepidermal blisters**, necrosis, and dermal papillary microabscesses; direct immunofluorescence studies reveal **granular deposits of IgA at tips of dermal papillae.**

case 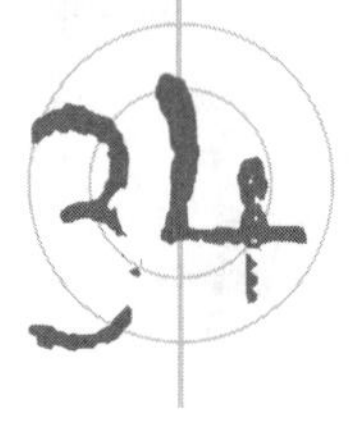

Dermatitis Herpetiformis

Differential

Erythema multiforme
Eczema
Scabies
Papular urticaria

Discussion

Dermatitis herpetiformis is a vesicular and extremely pruritic skin disease **associated with gluten sensitivity enteropathy** and IgA immune complexes deposited in dermal papillae; individuals with HLA-B8/DR-w3 haplotype are predisposed to developing the disease. **Males** are often more commonly affected, and peak incidence is in the third and fourth decades. Patients on long-term dapsone therapy should be monitored for hemolysis and methemoglobinemia.

Treatment

Dapsone therapy after confirming adequate glucose-6-phosphate dehydrogenase (G6PD) levels (dapsone produces hemolysis in G6PD-deficient individuals).

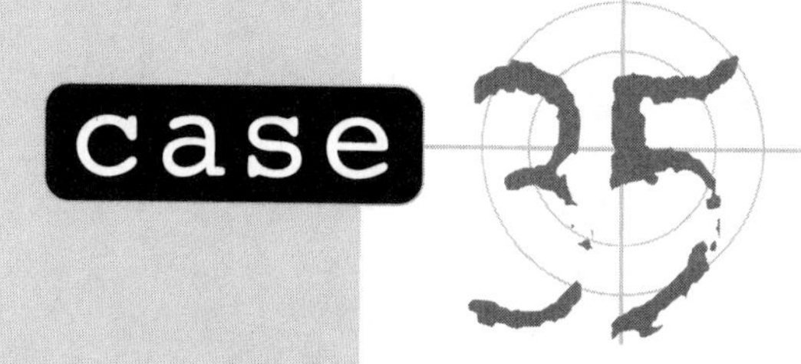

case 35

ID/CC A **16-year-old boy** complains of **multiple nevi** on her skin.

HPI She is concerned because an **aunt** who had a **similar illness** developed **malignant melanoma** and died of metastatic complications.

PE **Multiple nevi measuring 6 to 15 mm** noted; nevi are variegated shades of pink, tan, and brown and seen on back, chest, buttocks, scalp, and breasts; **borders are irregular** and **poorly defined** but lack the scalloping of malignant melanoma; no regional lymphadenopathy noted.

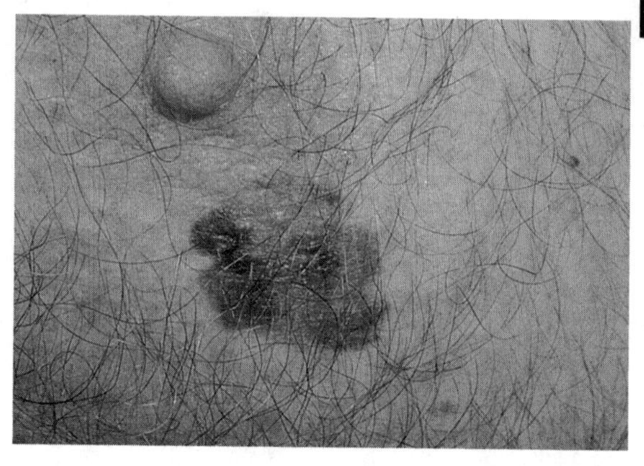

Figure 35-1. Asymmetric macule with irregular borders, variable color changes, and larger than 6 mm.

Micro Pathology Skin biopsy reveals melanocytes with **cytologic and architectural atypia**, enlarged and fused epidermal nevus cell nests, **lentiginous hyperplasia**, and **pigment incontinence**.

case 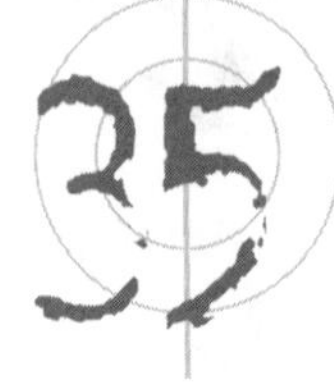

Dysplastic Nevus Syndrome

Differential

Malignant melanoma
Fibroma
Urticaria pigmentosum
Granuloma pyogenicum

Discussion

Dysplastic nevi are found in individuals with an autosomal dominant predisposition to develop acquired nevi; these **may develop into malignant melanoma.**

Treatment

Sun protection; regular skin exam to detect the development of malignant melanoma and for narrow-margin excisional biopsy of suspicious lesions. Family members should be regularly monitored.

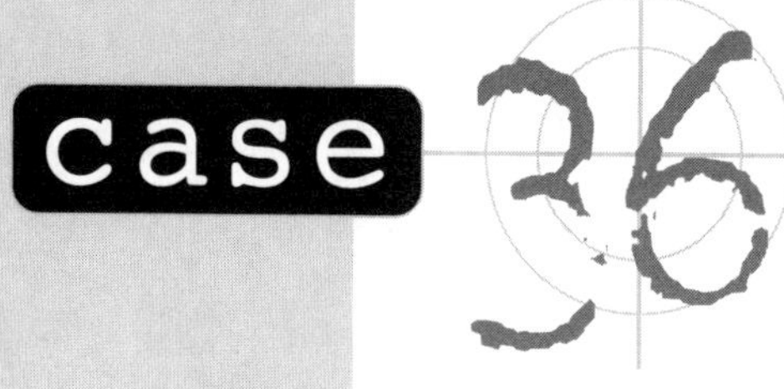

ID/CC A 24-year-old woman presents with a sudden-onset **skin rash** on both **forearms.**

HPI She suffers from **herpes labialis** and had a recent recurrence. Currently she is not taking any medications.

PE VS: normal. PE: **papulovesicular, erythematous skin lesions on both forearms,** occurring in **concentric rings with a clear center** (TARGET LESIONS); mucous membranes spared (vs. Stevens–Johnson syndrome).

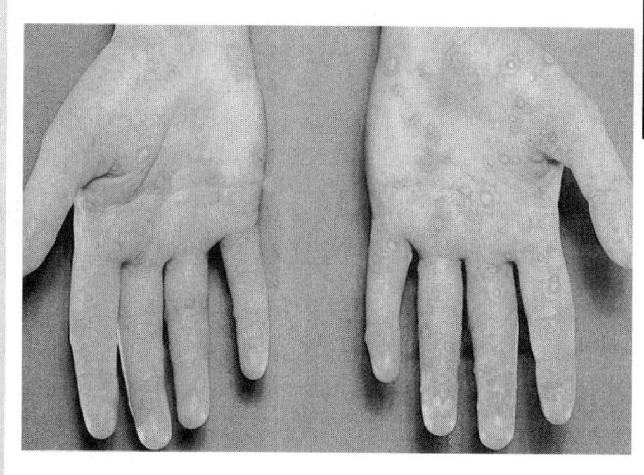

Figure 36-1. Multiple erythematous targetoid lesions on the palms.

Micro Pathology Skin biopsy reveals dermal edema and lymphocytic infiltrates intimately associated with degenerating keratinocytes along the dermal–epidermal junction; target lesions reveal a central necrosed area with a rim of perivenular inflammation.

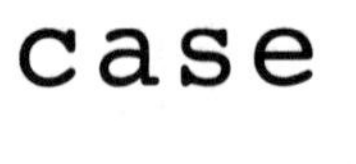
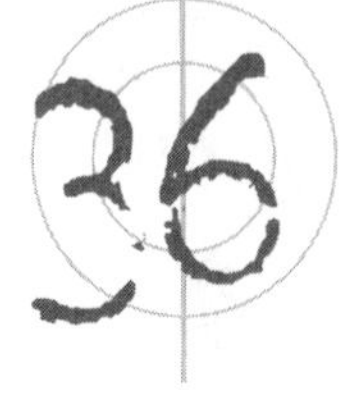

Erythema Multiforme

Differential

Bullous pemphigoid
Exfoliative dermatitis
Chemical burns
Scalded skin syndrome
Lyme disease

Discussion

Erythema multiforme is a hypersensitivity response to certain **drugs** (commonly sulfonamides, NSAIDs, penicillin, phenytoin) and **infections** (*Mycoplasma*, HSV). It is clinically divided into major and minor types. The minor type involves limited cutaneous surfaces, whereas the major type (STEVENS–JOHNSON SYNDROME) is characterized by toxic features and involvement of mucosal surfaces.

Treatment

Treat underlying cause, supportive therapy; **steroids** in severe cases.

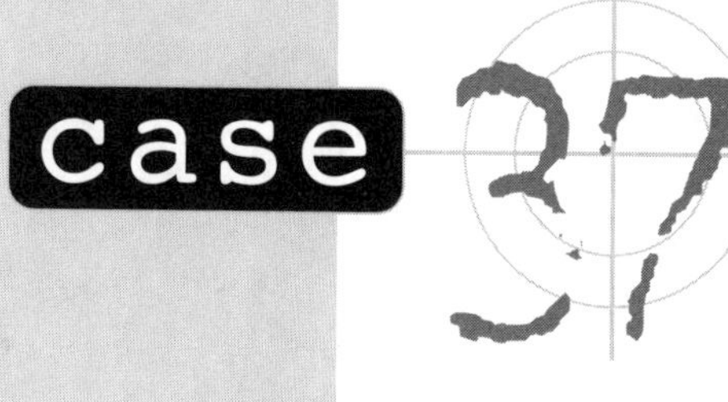

DERMATOLOGY

ID/CC A 24-year-old man presents with acute-onset, **painful swelling** in his **left axillae and chest.**

HPI He also reports fever and a history of poorly controlled juvenile-onset diabetes mellitus.

PE VS: fever (39°C); tachycardia (HR 110). PE: multiple, mobile, **extremely tender, erythematous, and fluctuant** axillary swellings; aspiration of swellings yields frank pus.

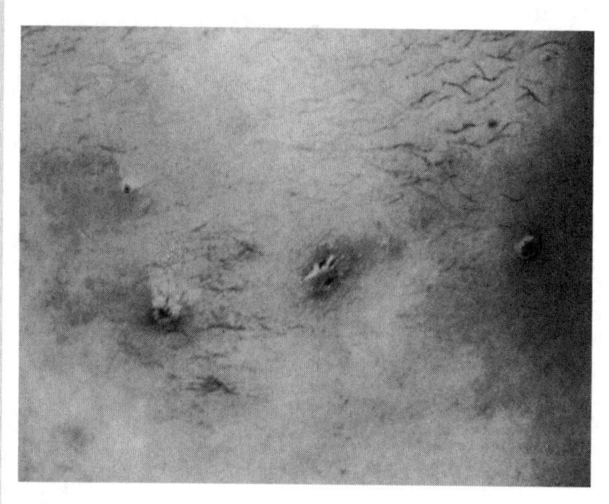

Figure 37-1. Multiple "boils" on the chest.

Labs CBC: **leukocytosis.** Gram stain of pus reveals Gram-positive cocci in clusters; culture grows coagulase-positive ***Staphylococcus aureus.***

case 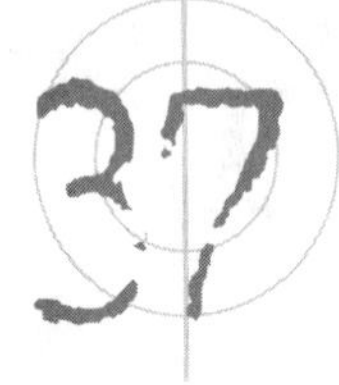

Furuncle

Differential

Carbuncle
Abscess
Folliculitis
Hidradenitis

Discussion

A boil (FURUNCLE) is a deep-seated infection of the hair follicle and adjacent subcutaneous tissue, most commonly occurring in moist hair-bearing parts of the body. **Diabetes, HIV,** and **IV drug abuse** are predisposing conditions. Recurrent cutaneous infections with ***S. aureus*** may occur due to a chronic carrier state (most commonly in the anterior nares).

Treatment

Incision and drainage; systemic antibiotics (empiric penicillinaseresistant β-lactams; then according to reported culture sensitivities).

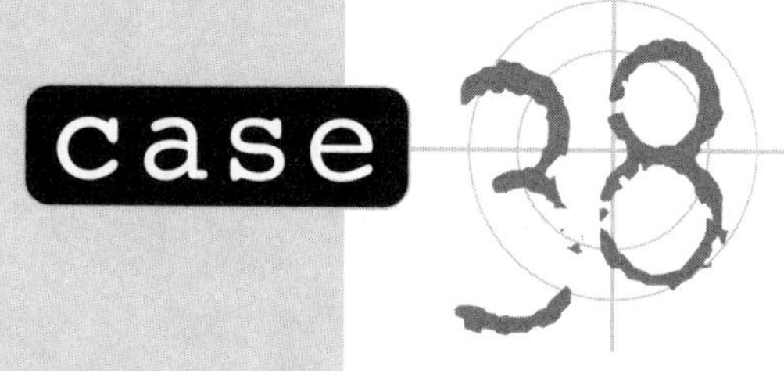

case 38

ID/CC A 23-year-old **HIV-positive** man presents with **nonpruritic reddish brown lesions.**

HPI He has had a continuous low-grade fever, significant weight loss over the past 6 months, and painless lumps in the cervical, axillary, and inguinal areas.

PE VS: fever. PE: emaciation; pallor; generalized lymphadenopathy; no hepatosplenomegaly or sternal tenderness; **reddish-purple plaques and nodules** over trunk and lower extremities; similar lesions noted in oral mucosa.

Labs ELISA/Western blot positive for HIV. CBC/PBS: **lymphocytopenia with depressed CD4 cell count** (<100).

Gross Pathology **Reddish-purple, raised plaques** and **firm nodules** with no suppuration.

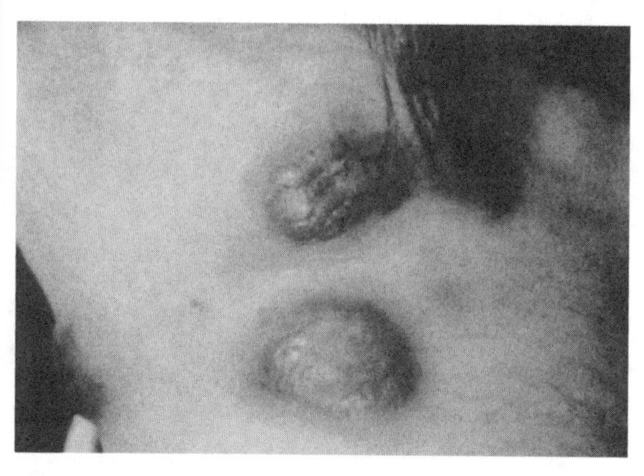

Figure 38-1. Reddish-purple plaques.

Micro Pathology Skin biopsy of nodular lesion shows malignant spindle cells with slitlike spaces containing RBCs, inflammatory cells, and hemosiderin-laden macrophages.

case 38

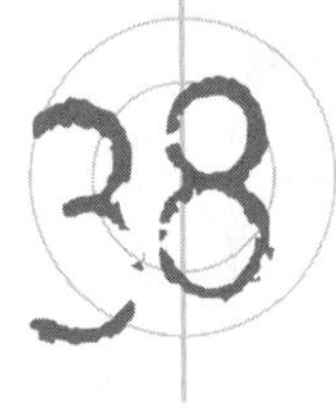

Kaposi Sarcoma

Differential

Bacillary angiomatosis
Hemangioma
Pyogenic granuloma
Purpura

Discussion

Kaposi sarcoma is the **most common cancer associated with AIDS** (epidemic type). The non-AIDS type affects Ashkenazi Jews (chronic or classic type) and Africans (lymphadenopathic or endemic type), but the disease is not as aggressive. **Human herpesvirus 8** is associated with all types; **disordered cytokine regulation** also plays a role. Other than the skin, lesions are most commonly found in the **lymph nodes, GI tract,** and **lung.** In contrast to lymphoma, lymphadenopathy presents early and is not significant.

Treatment

Radiation; chemotherapy with etoposide or doxorubicin, bleomycin, α-interferon, and vinblastine. If iatrogenic, stop immunosuppressive medication.

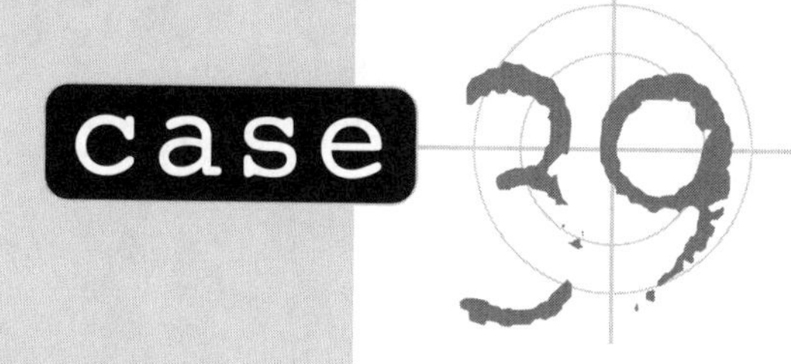

case 39

ID/CC A 4-year-old Japanese boy presents with **fever** and an **extensive skin rash.**

HPI A primary care physician had previously found the patient to have cervical adenitis; antibiotics were administered but achieved no response.

PE VS: fever. PE: **conjunctival congestion;** dry, red lips; **erythematous palms and soles;** indurative edema of peripheral extremities; **desquamation of fingertips;** various rashes of trunk; **cervical lymphadenopathy** >1.5 cm.

Labs **Throat swab and culture sterile.** CBC: routine blood counts normal; further differential blood counts reveal increased B-cell activation and T-helper-cell lymphocytopenia. Paul–Bunnell test for infectious mononucleosis negative; serologic tests rule out cytomegalovirus infection and toxoplasmosis.

Imaging Angio: presence of **coronary artery aneurysms.**

Gross Pathology Aneurismal dilatation of the coronary arteries.

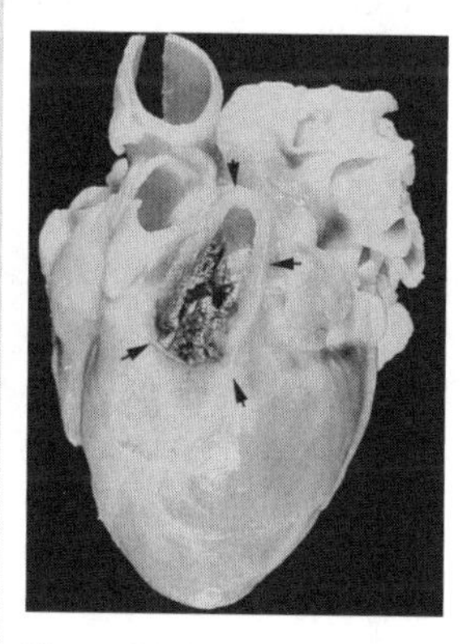

Figure 39-1. Coronary artery aneurysm with thrombosis.

Micro Pathology Coronary arteritis is usually demonstrated at autopsy together with aneurysm formation and thrombosis.

case 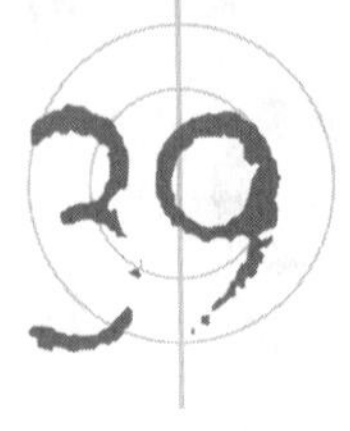

Kawasaki Syndrome

Differential

Acute rheumatic fever
Toxic shock syndrome
Measles
Drug reaction
Juvenile rheumatoid arthritis

Discussion

Kawasaki syndrome is usually self-limited, but in a few instances fatal coronary thrombosis has occurred during the acute stage of the disease or many months after apparently complete recovery. Case fatality rates have been about 1% to 2%.

Treatment

Aspirin and IV gamma globulin are effective in preventing coronary complications if initiated early.

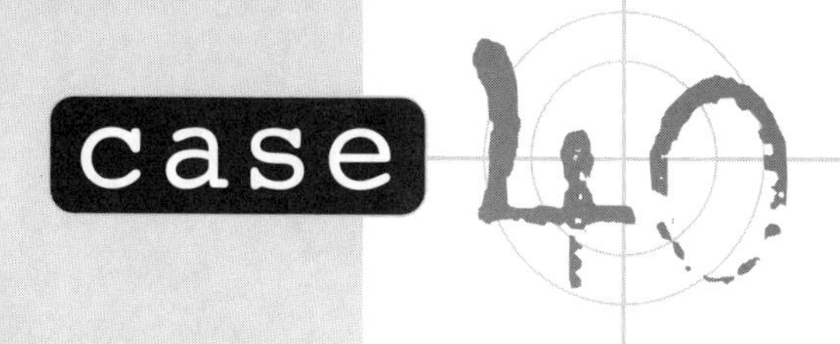

case 40

ID/CC A 30-year-old **woman** is seen with an **itchy rash** over her **wrists, forearms**, and **trunk.**

HPI She complains that fresh **lesions occur along scratch marks and areas of trauma** (KOEBNER PHENOMENON).

PE VS: no fever. PE: polygonal, **purple, flat-topped papules and plaques; tiny white dots and lines over papules** (WICKHAM STRIAE); white netlike pattern of **lesions over oral mucosa.**

Gross Pathology **Flat-topped, violaceous papules** and plaques **without scales.**

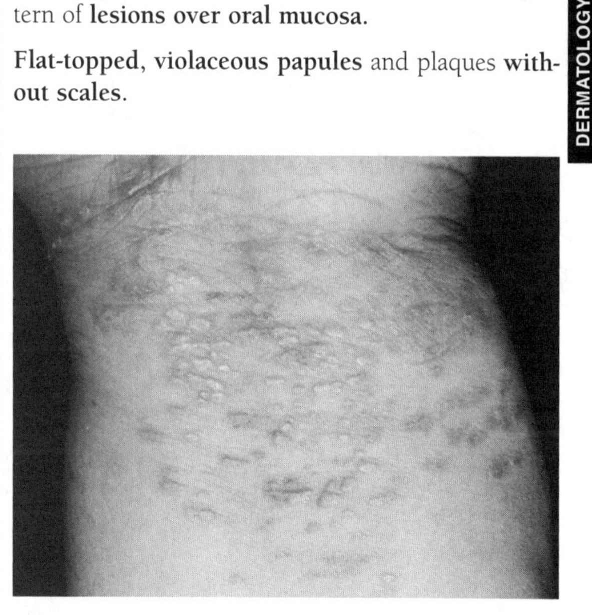

Figure 40-1. Persistently pruritic purplish, plane-topped, polygonal papules.

Micro Pathology Dense, **bandlike (lichenoid) lymphocytic infiltrate** (predominantly T cells) along the dermal–epidermal junction; **sawtooth pattern of rete ridges**; destruction of basal cells.

case 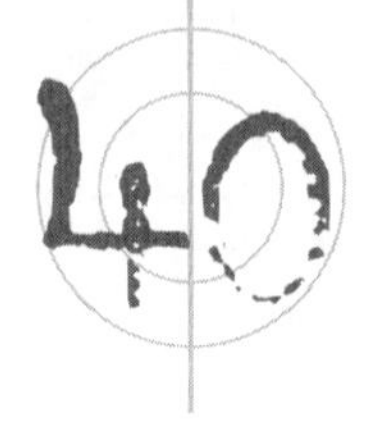

Lichen Planus

Differential

Pityriasis rosea
Psoriasis
Syphilis
Tinea corporis

Discussion

Lichen planus is a **self-limited inflammatory skin** disease, but in some cases it may be present for several years. Females are affected more frequently than males. Postinflammatory hyperpigmentation may be evident after the lesions subside. Medications such as tetracycline, penicillamine, and hydrochlorothiazide can cause lichen planus–like skin reactions.

Treatment

Steroids, topical (potent fluorinated) or systemic; psoralens with UVA therapy in refractory cases.

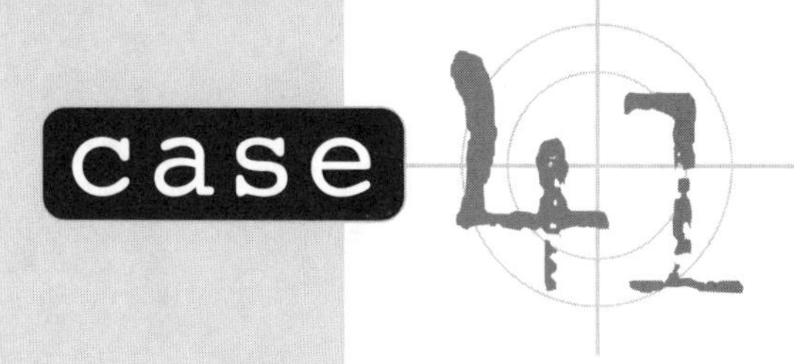

case 41

ID/CC A 50-year-old **white** man presents with an itchy, **rapidly enlarging, pigmented lesion** on the sole of his left foot.

HPI He states that the spot has **recently changed color** dramatically; once lightly pigmented, it is now a deep purple hue.

PE **Irregular, asymmetric, deeply pigmented lesion with various shades** of red and blue; diameter **>6 mm;** left-sided nontender **inguinal lymphadenopathy.**

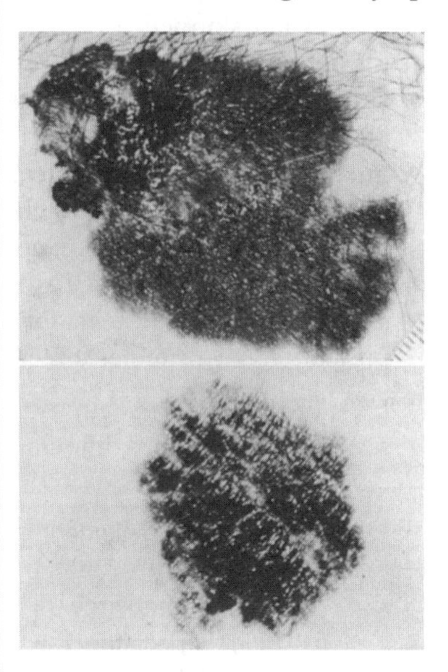

Figure 41-1. Irregular, asymmetric, deeply pigmented lesion.

Gross Pathology **Slightly raised;** deeply pigmented with uneven hues and irregular border.

Micro Pathology Excisional biopsy shows tumor-free borders along with large, atypical, variably pigmented cells with irregular nuclei and eosinophilic nucleoli in epidermis and papillary dermis; dermal invasion noted in some places; metastases shown on lymph node biopsy.

case 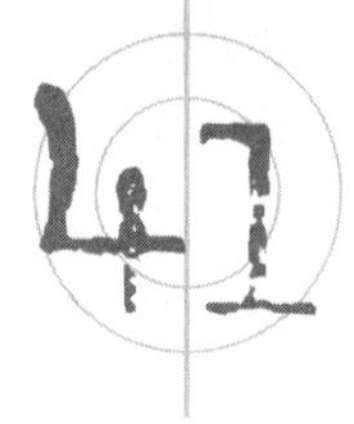

Malignant Melanoma

Differential

Blue nevi
Cherry angiomata
Spitz nevi
Squamous cell carcinoma
Dysplastic nevi

Discussion

Of all skin cancers, melanoma is responsible for the largest number of deaths. An increased incidence is seen in **fair-skinned** people and in those with **dysplastic nevi, immunosuppression**, and **excessive sun exposure.** Melanomas undergo a **radial** (superficial) **growth** phase followed by an invasive, **vertical growth** phase. **Bleeding, ulceration**, and **pain are late manifestations.** The **chance of metastasis increases with depth of invasion** (measured using Clark levels I–V). Metastatic melanomas are **incurable** and signify the **need for early detection** and prevention (e.g., sunblock, clothing).

Treatment

Excision with wide margin, regional lymph node dissection, chemotherapy, immunotherapy.

Breakout Point

The ABCDE of malignant melanoma
A Asymmetry
B Border irregularity
C Color variegation
D Diameter
E Evolving

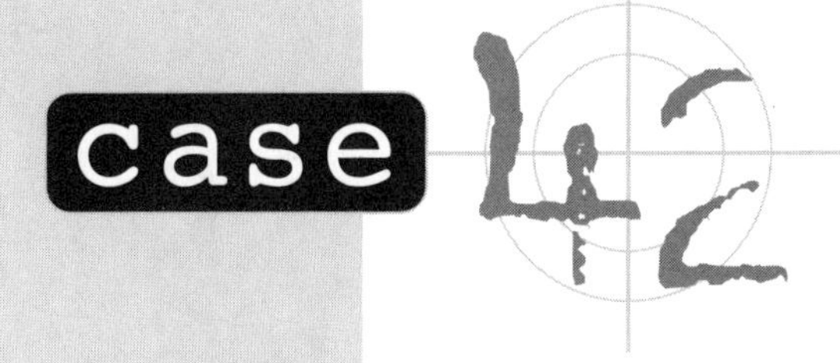

ID/CC A 60-year-old man presents with multiple lumps and a **chronic**, pruritic, erythematous **rash** that has spread and now **involves almost his entire body.**

HPI He has seen many doctors, but the rash **has not responded to** a variety of medications, including **topical and systemic steroids.**

PE Erythematous, circinate rash in **plaques** with **exfoliation** (SCALING); some **nodules** seen on face, trunk, lower abdomen, and buttocks.

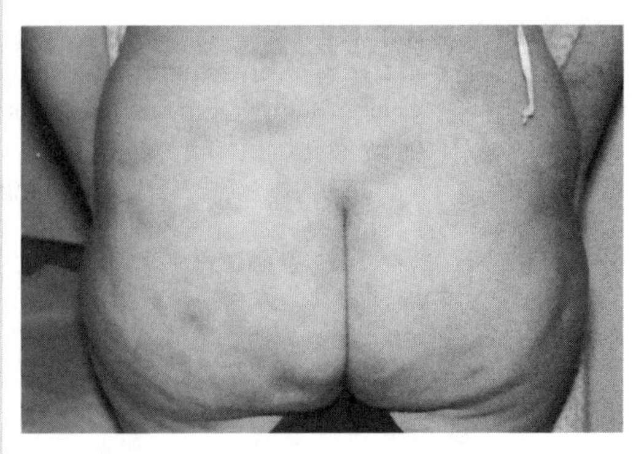

Figure 42-1. Characteristic "smudgy," poorly defined patches and plaques in a typical location.

Labs CBC/PBS: lymphocytosis. Atypical. **PAS-positive, large, CD4-antigen-positive** (helper T-cell) **lymphocytes with characteristic multiconvoluted, "cerebriform" nuclei** (SÉZARY–LUTZNER CELLS).

Imaging CXR: no mediastinal lymphadenopathy.

Gross Pathology Reddish-brown, **kidney-shaped plaques** (vs. Hodgkin lymphoma); hence name **"red man's disease"**; exfoliation, nodule formation, and sometimes ulceration.

Micro Pathology Dermal infiltration with exocytosis of atypical mononuclear cells within epidermis found singly or within punched-out **epidermal microabscesses** (PAUTRIER ABSCESSES).

case 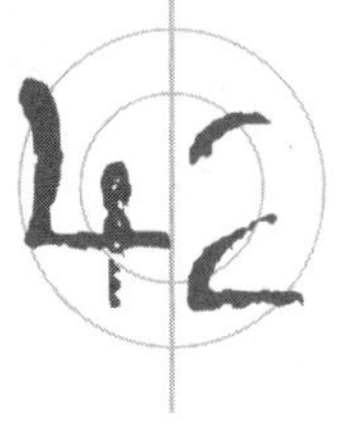

Mycosis Fungoides

Differential

Diffuse large cell lymphoma

Eczema

Drug reaction

Atopic dermatitis

Discussion

Mycosis fungoides is a malignant cutaneous helper T-cell lymphoma; disseminated disease with exfoliative dermatitis and generalized lymphadenopathy is termed **Sézary syndrome.**

Treatment

Topical treatment employing PUVA; total skin electron-beam therapy; prednisone and topical chemotherapy; for advanced disease, systemic treatment with interferon, retinoids, photopheresis, and systemic chemotherapy with single agents.

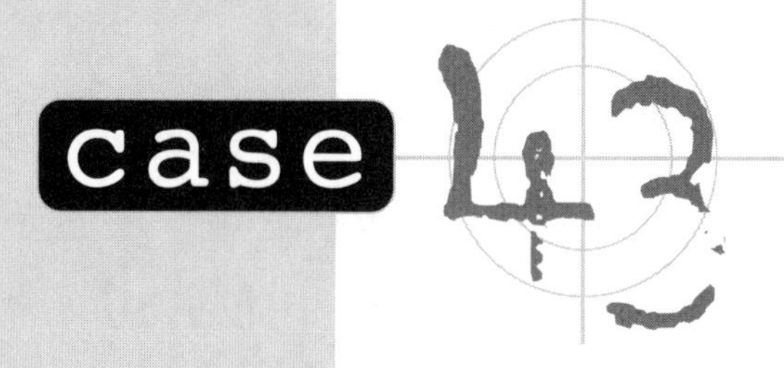

case 43

ID/CC A 25-year-old man is admitted to the hospital for an evaluation of **recurrent epistaxis.**

HPI The patient's mother died of a **massive pulmonary hemorrhage due to an arteriovenous malformation.**

PE **Small telangiectatic lesions** seen on lips, oral and nasal mucosa, tongue, and tips of fingers and toes; anemia noted; no pulmonary bruit heard (to detect an AV malformation).

DERMATOLOGY

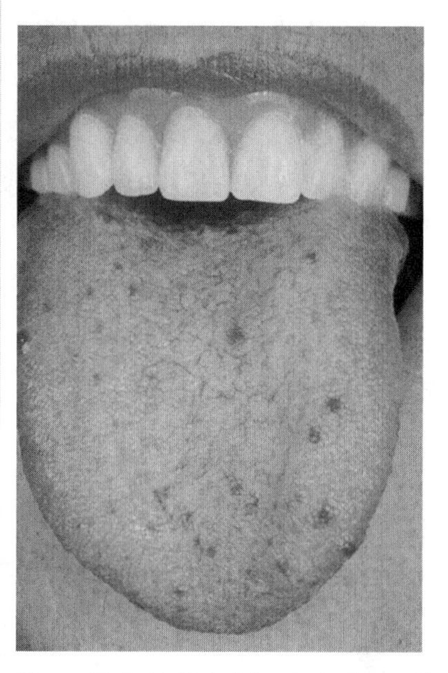

Figure 43-1. Multiple telangiectasias on the tongue.

Labs CBC: normocytic, normochromic anemia (due to occult gastrointestinal blood loss). Guaiac positive.

Imaging MR: AV malformations in liver and spleen.

Micro Pathology Irregularly dilated capillaries and venules.

case 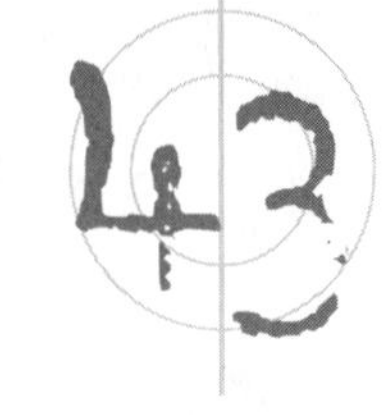

Osler–Weber–Rendu Syndrome

Differential

Ataxia telangiectasia
Acne rosacea
Dermatomyositis
Scleroderma

Discussion

Hereditary hemorrhagic telangiectasia, or Osler–Weber–Rendu syndrome, is inherited as an **autosomal dominant trait**. Telangiectasias may first be seen during adolescence and then increase in incidence with age, peaking between the ages of 45 and 60 years. AV fistulas may present with hemoptysis, indicating high morbidity.

Treatment

Nasal packing, **cautery**, and **estrogens** may be tried to control recurrent epistaxis; significant visceral AV malformations may require embolization.

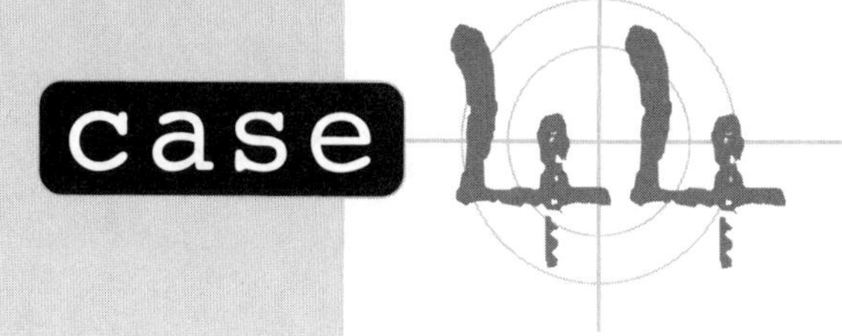

case 44

ID/CC A **45-year-old woman** visits her dermatologist complaining of **painful, blistering skin lesions over her back, chest, and arms that break down and leave denuded skin areas.**

HPI Over the past few years she has had **large recurrent aphthous ulcers in the mouth.** She was not taking any drugs before her symptoms developed.

PE **Large aphthous ulcers** seen over oral and vaginal mucosa; **vesiculobullous skin lesions** seen in **various stages**; vertical pressure over bullae leads to **lateral extension** ("BULLA SPREAD SIGN"); skin over bullae **peels like that of a "hot tomato"** (NIKOLSKY SIGN).

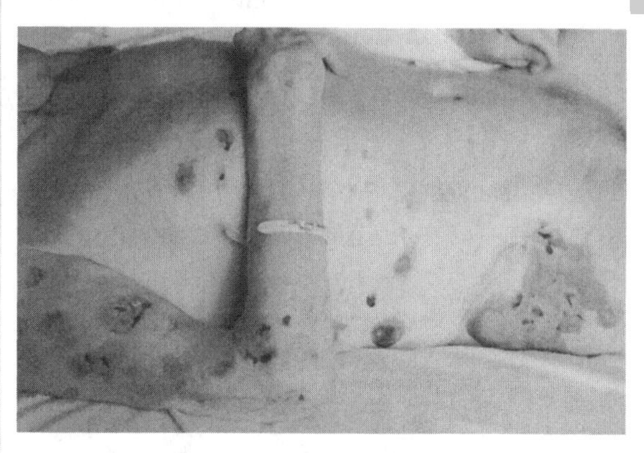

Figure 44-1. Flaccid bullae and erosions.

Labs Indirect immunofluorescence test to detect antibodies in serum shows presence of IgG antibodies.

Gross Pathology Fresh vesicle is selected for biopsy.

Micro Pathology Lesions show **loss of cohesion of epidermal cells** (ACANTHOLYSIS) that produces clefts directly above basal cell layer; **direct immunofluorescence** reveals **characteristic IgG intercellular staining** and **deposits.**

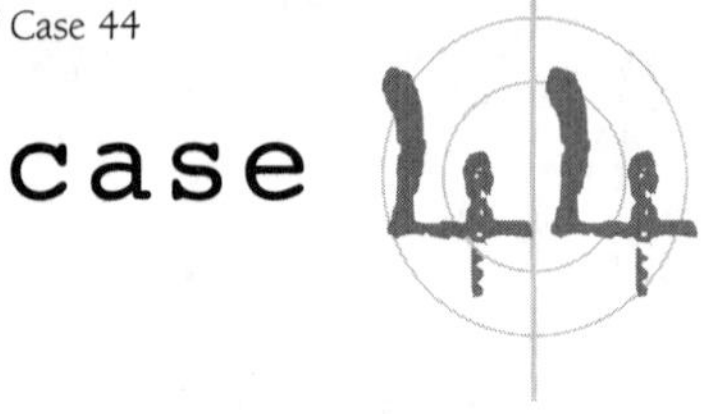

Pemphigus

Differential

Bullous pemphigoid
Dermatitis herpetiformis
Erythema multiforme
Aphthous ulcers
Herpetic stomatitis

Discussion

Pemphigus vulgaris, an intraepidermal blistering disease of the skin and mucous membranes, usually appears in individuals in the third to fifth decade of life. The blisters result from loss of adhesion between epidermal cells caused by the production of autoantibodies that are directed against keratinocyte cell surface proteins; loss of cell–cell contact between desmosomes (which are sites of attachment for epidermal cells) has been demonstrated by electron microscopy. Untreated pemphigus vulgaris is often fatal.

Treatment

Steroids are mainstay of therapy; cytotoxic drugs (cyclophosphamide).

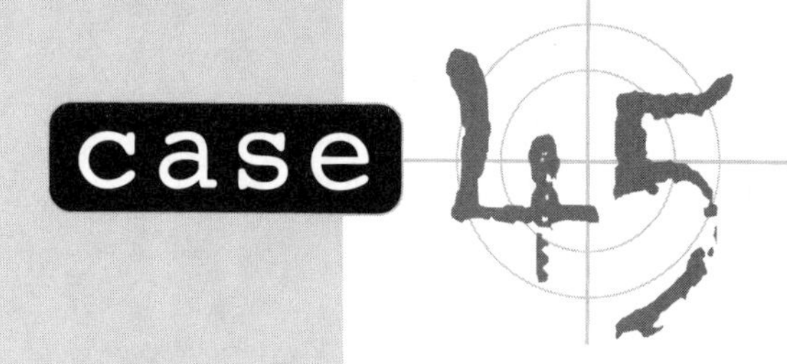

DERMATOLOGY

ID/CC A 17-year-old girl presents with a **scaly rash** on her **trunk.**

HPI Three weeks ago, she noticed a small scaly rash on her neck that progressed in about a week to involve the trunk and upper extremities. Aside from the rash, she is asymptomatic. She is sexually active.

PE VS: normal. PE: crop of **oval, erythematous, scaly maculopapular lesions** on trunk, neck, and proximal extremities in a **"Christmas tree" distribution.**

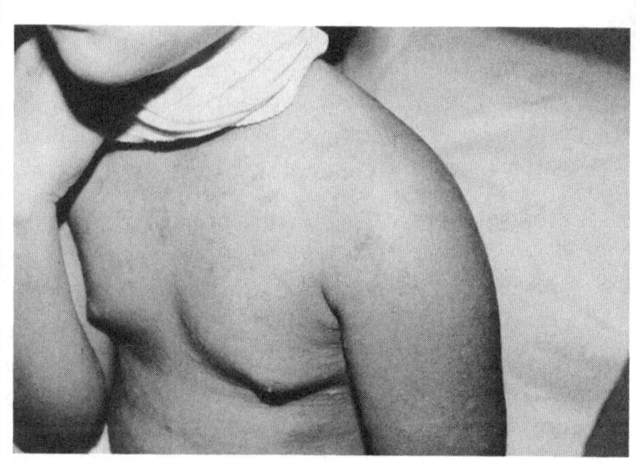

Figure 45-1. Circular and ovoid papules and plaques with scaling on the trunk and proximal extremities.

Labs RPR/VDRL non-reactive; ELISA for HIV negative.

Gross Pathology Biopsy specimen shows **superficial perivascular dermatitis.**

case 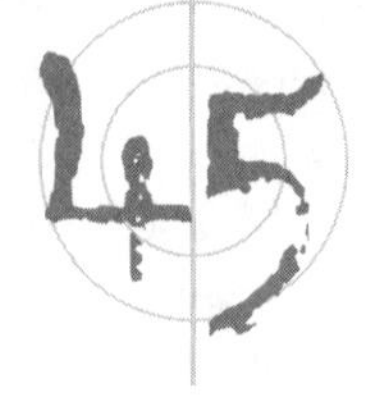

Pityriasis Rosea

Differential

Syphilis
Drug eruption
Eczema
Tinea corporis
Viral exanthem

Discussion

Pityriasis rosea is a common skin rash with the highest incidence in young adults and teenagers. The disease is twice as common in women as in men. In most cases, the initial lesion is a 1- to 10-cm, oval maculopapular lesion, called a "**herald patch,**" that is commonly found on the trunk or neck. Pityriasis rosea is a clinical diagnosis; it is important to differentiate the disease from **secondary syphilis, tinea versicolor, psoriasis**, and **drug reactions.**

Treatment

Treat with **moisturizers** and **antipruritic lotions; topical steroids** or **oral antihistamines** rarely required; **ultraviolet B light** used to relieve pruritus in resistant cases; provide reassurance, as disease is **benign and self-limited**, and **recurrence** is **uncommon.**

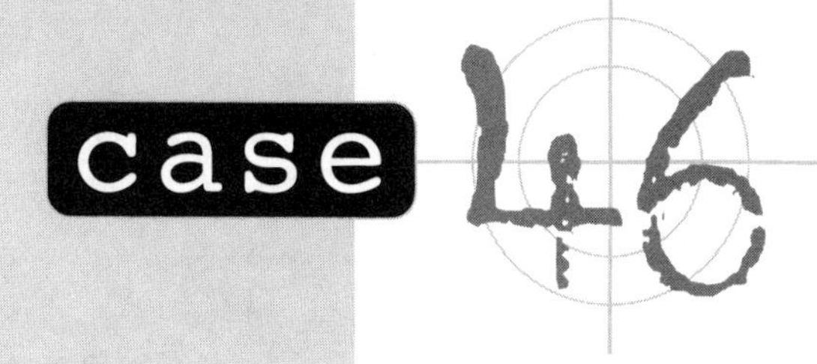

case 46

ID/CC A 40-year-old man comes to a dermatology outpatient clinic with an extensive, mildly pruritic, and chronic skin rash.

HPI **It improves during the summer and markedly worsens in cold weather.** The patient was previously diagnosed by an orthopaedic surgeon with **distal interphalangeal joint arthropathy.**

PE Multiple **salmon-colored plaques** with **overlying silvery scales** seen over back and extensor aspects of upper and lower limbs; on removing scale, **underlying pinpoint bleeding capillaries** seen (AUSPITZ SIGN); lesions seen along scratch marks (KOEBNER PHENOMENA); **pitting of nails** with occasional onycholysis seen.

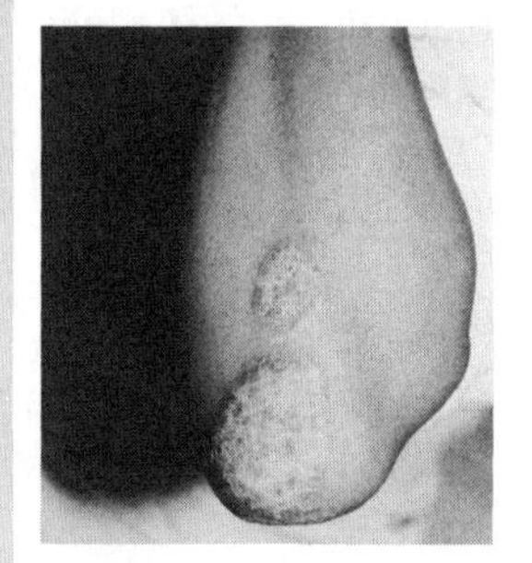

Figure 46-1. Well-defined erythematous, scaling plaques on the extensor surface of the arm in a patient.

Imaging XR, hands: asymmetric degenerative changes involving the distal interphalangeal joints, with "**pencil-in-cup**" deformity.

Micro Pathology Skin biopsy reveals markedly thickened stratum corneum with layered zones of parakeratosis (retention of nuclei); markedly hyperplastic epidermis with elongation of rete projections; collections of PMNs within the stratum corneum (MUNRO MICROABSCESSES); **marked degree of epidermal hyperplasia with little inflammatory infiltrate** (characteristic microscopic finding).

case 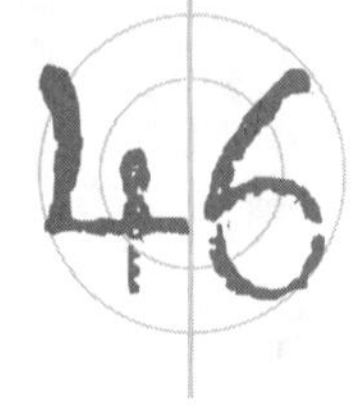

Psoriasis

Differential

Atopic dermatitis
Contact dermatitis
Pityriasis rosea
Tinea

Discussion

Psoriasis is a hereditary condition that is characterized by well-defined plaques covered by silvery scales. Lesions are most commonly seen in an extensor distribution, but the nails, scalp, palms, and soles may also be involved; arthritis of the distal interphalangeal joint may be seen in 20% of cases. Parenteral corticosteroids are contraindicated owing to the possibility of inducing pustular lesions.

Treatment

Exposure to sunlight. The following have been used either alone or in combination: occlusive dressings, tar ointment, dithranol, PUVA, topical steroids, and cytotoxic drugs such as methotrexate.

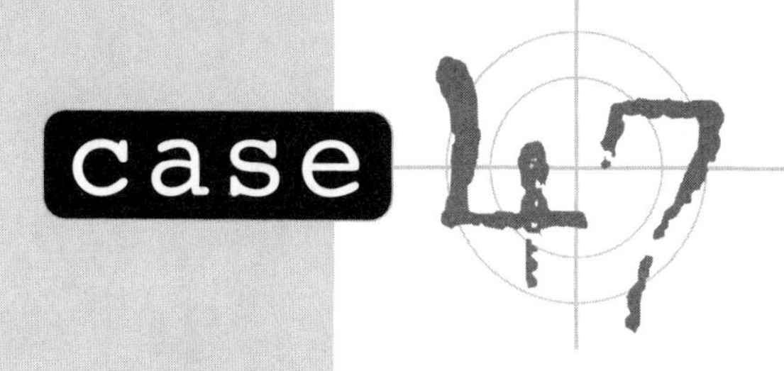

case 47

ID/CC A **40-year-old woman presents** with an extremely painful **ulcer** on her left **calf.**

HPI The lesion appeared a month ago as a **small boil** after the patient hurt herself. It then became progressively larger until it cracked open 2 days ago. The patient reports a history of **ulcerative colitis,** which was diagnosed several years ago and managed effectively with steroid enemas and oral sulfasalazine.

PE VS: normal. PE: 10- by 10-cm deep **ulcer with violaceous border** overhanging ulcer bed; no lymphadenopathy; good distal pulses palpable.

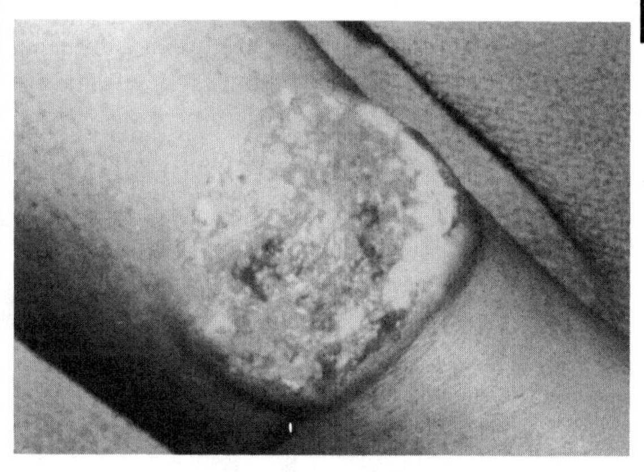

Figure 47-1. Ulcer with violaceous border.

Labs No growth demonstrated on Gram stain and culture of wound swab; **skin biopsy diagnostic.**

Micro Pathology Skin biopsy reveals hyperkeratosis; dermal perivascular round cell infiltration, and mixed infiltrate (neutrophils, lymphocytes, macrophages) extending to the subcutaneous plane.

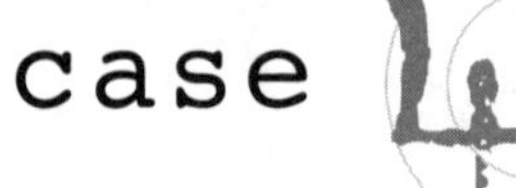
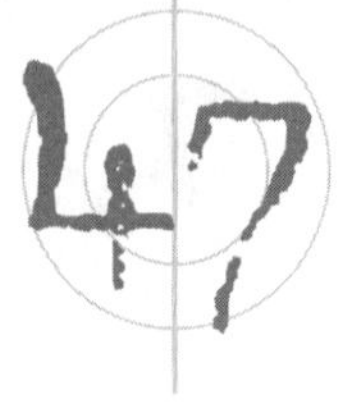

Pyoderma Gangrenosum

Differential

Insect bite
Ecthyma gangrenosum
Impetigo
Sporotrichosis
Venous insufficiency

Discussion

Commonly associated conditions include **inflammatory bowel disease** and **leukemia** or **preleukemic states** (usually myelocytic leukemia or monoclonal gammopathies). Most cases occur in the fourth or fifth decades of life, with females affected slightly more often than males.

Treatment

Systemic **steroids** (oral prednisone or IV pulse methylprednisone) and **immunosuppressive** therapy (cyclosporine or tacrolimus); antibiotics for secondary infection and narcotic analgesics for pain.

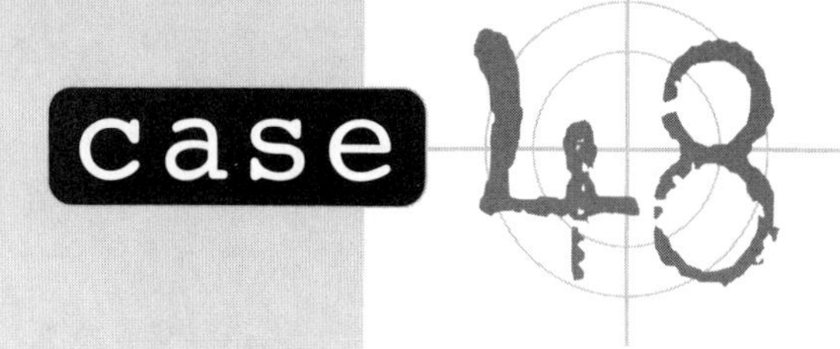

case 48

ID/CC A 40-year-old white man presents with a **scaly, mildly pruritic rash over the face and scalp.**

HPI He reports that the rash is **aggravated by humidity, scratching, emotional stress, and seasonal changes.** He tested **HIV positive** last year and has since maintained a good CD4 count without any antiretroviral therapy.

PE VS: normal. PE: interspersed thick **adherent crusts and scales** overlying areas of **greasy, yellow-red inflamed skin** involving the **scalp, forehead, nasolabial folds,** and **chest.**

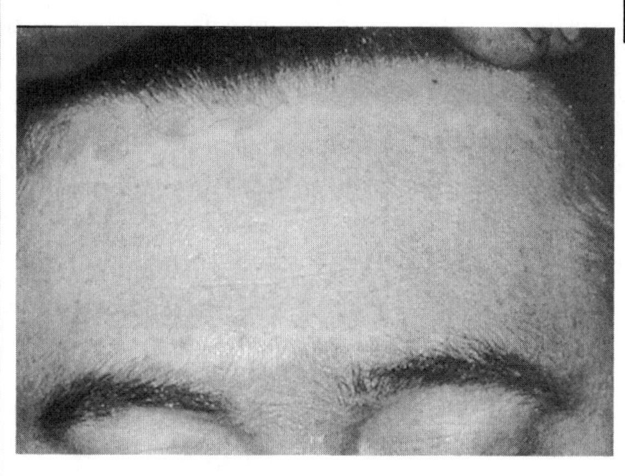

Figure 48-1. Greasy, yellow-red inflamed skin involving the scalp.

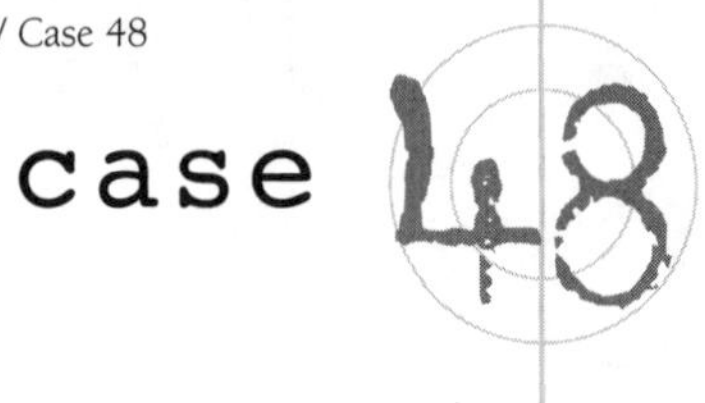

Seborrheic Dermatitis

Differential

Atopic dermatitis
Drug-induced photosensitivity
Rosacea
Tinea capitis
Contact dermatitis

Discussion

A papulosquamous skin rash involving areas rich in sebaceous glands; seborrheic dermatitis is thought to result from an abnormal host immune response toward a common skin commensal, ***Pityrosporum ovale.*** Various drugs (haloperidol, lithium, methyldopa, cimetidine) may worsen the condition. It is also commonly found in patients suffering from parkinsonism and in those recovering from an acute MI.

Treatment

Maintain **good hygiene; medicated shampoo; topical hydrocortisone lotion** or ketoconazole cream.

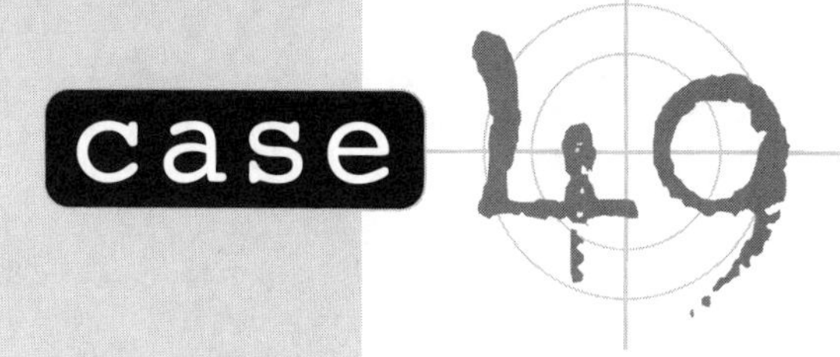

ID/CC A 6-year-old white girl is brought to the ER by her mother because of severe **itching, joint pain**, and a **generalized skin eruption.**

HPI She had received an **injection of penicillin 6 days before** for streptococcal tonsillitis. Her mother denies any relevant past medical history, including allergies. Once in the hospital, the child developed fever, **edema** of the ankles and knees, hematuria, and lethargy.

PE VS: fever. PE: generalized **urticarial skin rash;** axillary and inguinal lymphadenopathy; splenomegaly; redness and swelling of knees and ankles.

Labs Increased ESR; decreased C3, C4 levels. UA: proteinuria; hematuria.

Gross Pathology Generalized wheals throughout body.

Micro Pathology Vascular lesions show fibrinoid necrosis and a neutrophilic infiltrate; **immune complex deposition in kidney and joints.**

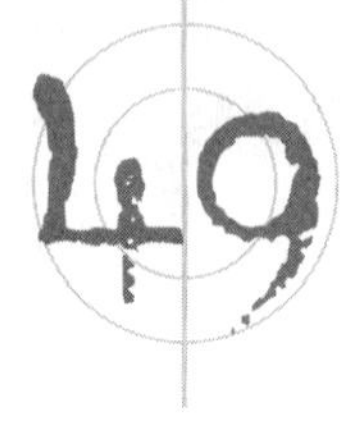

Serum Sickness

Differential

Cryoglobulinemia
Systemic lupus erythematosus
Dermatitis herpetiformis
Erythema multiforme

Discussion

Serum sickness is a **type III hypersensitivity reaction** (immune complex disease) with a latency period between exposure to the offending agent (drugs, serum) and the appearance of signs and symptoms; it is usually self-limiting.

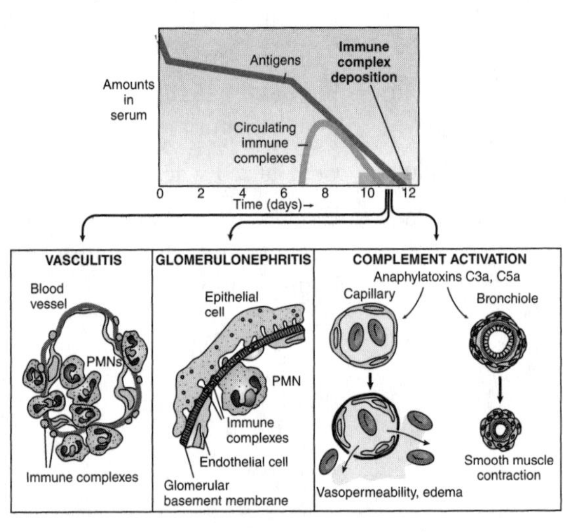

Figure 49-1. Type III hypersensitivity.

Discussion

In the serum sickness model of immune complex tissue injury, antibody is produced against a circulating antigen, and immune complexes form in the blood. These complexes deposit in tissues such as blood vessels and glomeruli and, augmented by complement activation, induce tissue injury or dysfunctional responses.

Treatment

Antihistamines; corticosteroids; aspirin; epinephrine if severe.

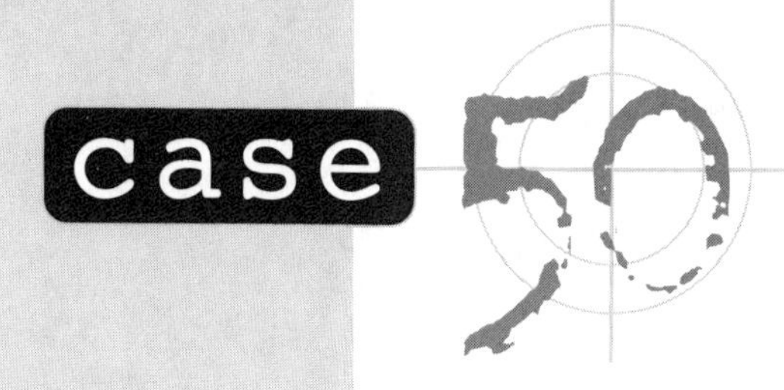

case 50

ID/CC An 8-year-old **black boy** complains of **unsightly white** (depigmented) **patches** on his knees, elbows (bony prominences), and buttocks.

HPI He has no history of associated **pruritus** or **discomfort.** The first patch appeared over the left elbow a few months ago, and the process has been **progressive** since then.

PE PE: flat, well-demarcated areas of **depigmentation** on face (perioral or periocular), elbows, knees, and neck and in skin folds; sites of recent skin trauma are also seen to have **undergone depigmentation** (KOEBNER PHENOMENON); **most hairs within vitiliginous patch are white.**

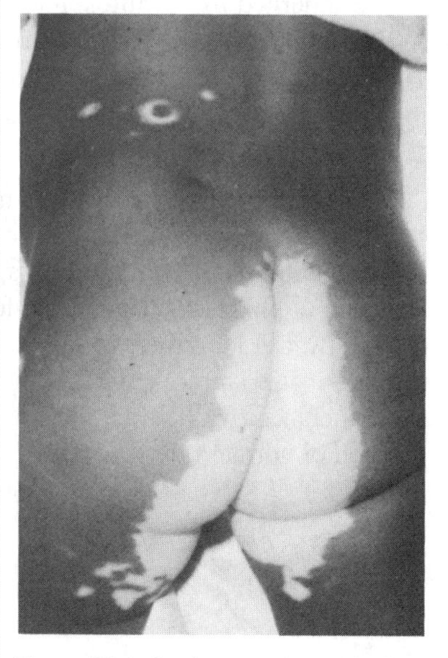

Figure 50-1. Depigmentation with distinct borders.

Micro Pathology **Absent melanin pigment** on skin biopsy stain with ferric ferricyanide; **absence of melanocytes** on electron microscopy.

case 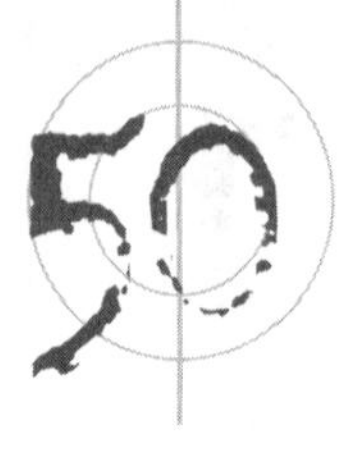

Vitiligo

Differential

Tinea versicolor
Nevus depigmentosus
Leprosy
Hypothyroidism

Discussion

Vitiligo usually appears in otherwise-healthy persons, but several systemic disorders occur more often in patients with vitiligo, including thyroid disease (e.g., hyperthyroidism, Graves' disease, and thyroiditis), Addison disease, pernicious anemia, alopecia areata, uveitis, and diabetes mellitus. Precipitating factors such as illness, emotional stress, or physical trauma are often associated with its onset. The disease may be inherited as an **autosomal dominant trait** with incomplete penetrance and variable expression. Most studies, however, point to an **autoimmune** basis (circulating complement-binding antimelanocyte antibodies have been detected).

Treatment

No established satisfactory treatment exists, although sunscreens protect and limit the tanning of normally pigmented skin. A promising approach is oral psoralen (a photosensitizing drug) followed by exposure to artificial long-wave ultraviolet light (UVA); potent fluorinated topical steroids may also be helpful. Generalized vitiligo may be treated by depigmentation of normal skin.

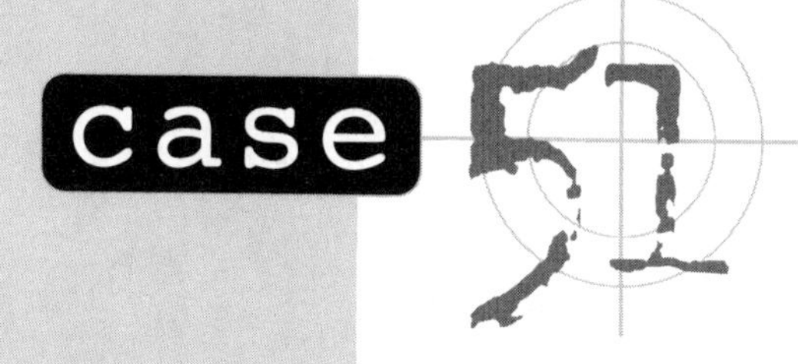

case 51

ID/CC A 17-year-old white boy undergoing chemotherapy for disseminated Hodgkin lymphoma complains of severe headaches, nausea, and weight loss.

HPI The patient had been on **aminoglycosides.** When questioned, he is uncertain of place and time, but despite his confusion he describes his urine as appearing reddish orange over the past few weeks.

PE Confused but alert; underweight; no acute distress.

Labs Lytes: increased potassium. UA: hematuria; mild proteinuria; granular casts in urine; renal tubular epithelial cells in sediment; isotonic urine osmolality; **elevated urinary sodium** (>40 mEq/L). Increased serum inorganic phosphorus; **azotemia** with BUN/creatinine ratio of 5 (within normal limits); fractional excretion of sodium >1%.

Gross Pathology Kidneys enlarged, flabby, and pale with edema.

Micro Pathology Necrosis of tubular epithelial cells that slough into lumen, forming casts and causing blockade; hydropic degeneration of epithelium.

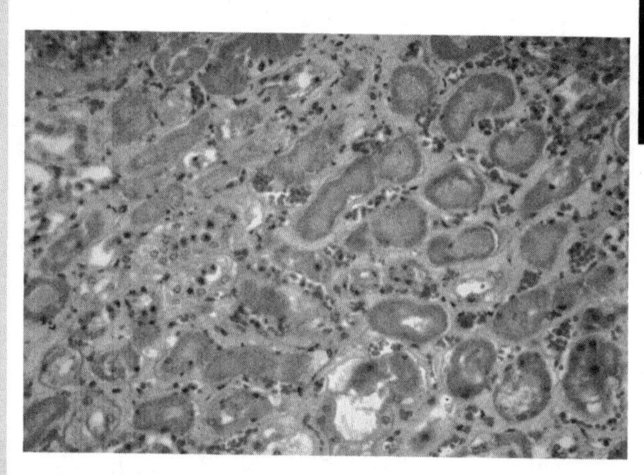

Figure 51-1. Necrosis of tubular epithelial cells lacking nuclei with sloughing into the tubular lumen.

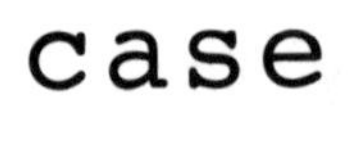
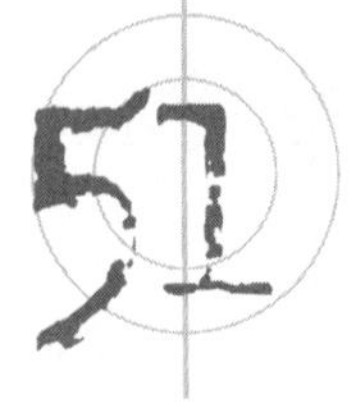

Acute Tubular Necrosis

Differential

Azotemia
Chronic renal failure
Acute glomerulonephritis
Interstitial nephritis
Renal vasculitis

Discussion

Acute tubular necrosis is defined as acute tubular damage resulting in acute renal failure; it is caused by prolonged ischemia or toxins (nephrotoxic drugs) and is usually reversible, as long as the epithelial basement membrane remains intact.

Treatment

Discontinue offending agent; fluid and electrolyte management; renal replacement therapy with hemodialysis if indicated.

case 52

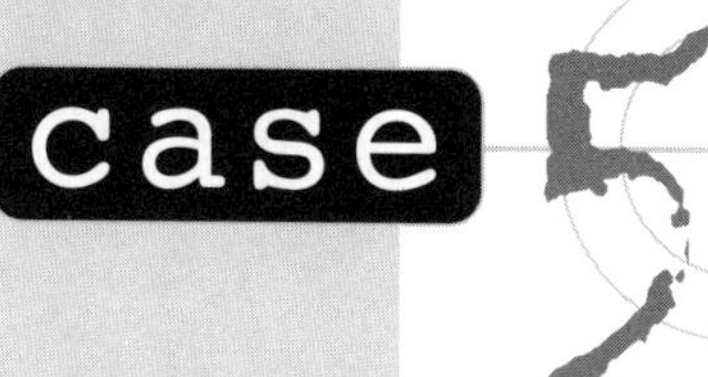

ID/CC	A 47-year-old white man enters the emergency room complaining of a sudden-onset, **severe headache** that is the "**worst headache of his life.**"
HPI	He also describes slow-onset dull pain in his left flank and blood in his urine. He was recently treated for **recurrent UTIs**, which were attributed to an enlarged prostate gland. His **father** died of **chronic renal failure**, and his paternal **grandfather** died of **cerebral hemorrhage.**
PE	VS: hypertension (BP 170/110). PE: palpable, nontender **abdominal mass** on both flanks; nuchal rigidity.
Labs	UA: albuminuria; microscopic **hematuria** (no WBCs or casts). Slightly increased BUN, creatinine.
Imaging	Angio, neuro: ruptured **berry aneurysm.** CT/US, abdomen: **multiple kidney and liver cysts.**
Gross Pathology	Kidneys markedly enlarged and heavy with hundreds of cysts that almost replace normal parenchyma; cysts thick walled, ranging from a few millimeters to several centimeters in diameter.

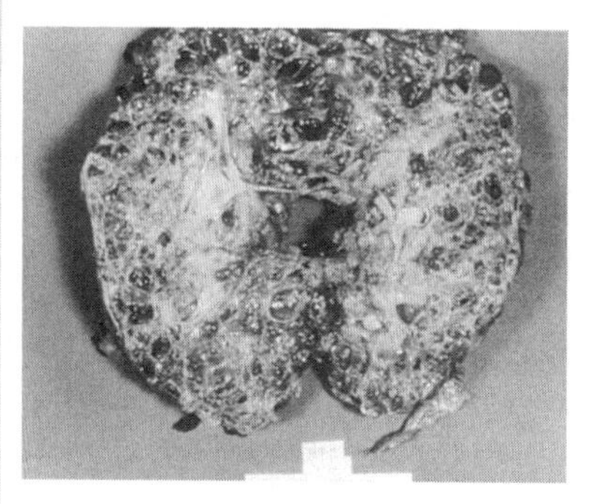

Figure 52-1. Extensive parenchymal replacement by cortical and medullary cysts of varying sizes.

Micro Pathology	Cystic dilatation of tubules; epithelial cell hyperplasia; cuboidal epithelium lining cysts.

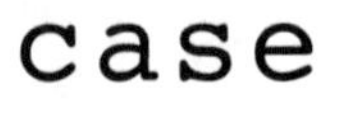
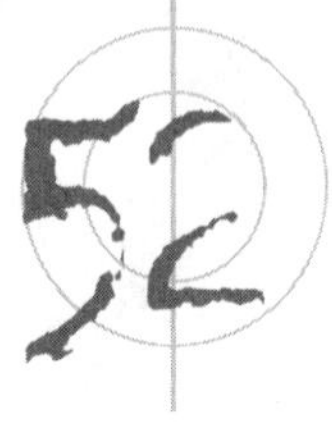

Adult Polycystic Kidney Disease

Differential

Autosomal recessive polycystic kidney disease
Medullary cystic disease
Renal dysplasia
Von Hippel–Lindau syndrome

Discussion

Adult polycystic kidney disease (APKD) is an **autosomal dominant** disease caused by a defect in **chromosome 16** in which the renal parenchyma is converted to hundreds of fluid-filled cysts, resulting in progressive renal failure in adulthood. Cysts may also involve the pancreas, liver, lungs, and spleen. It is associated with berry aneurysms of the circle of Willis, hypertension, and mitral valve prolapse. Unlike most autosomal dominant disorders, this disease does not manifest until later in life.

Treatment

Aneurysm "clipping"; dialysis and renal transplantation.

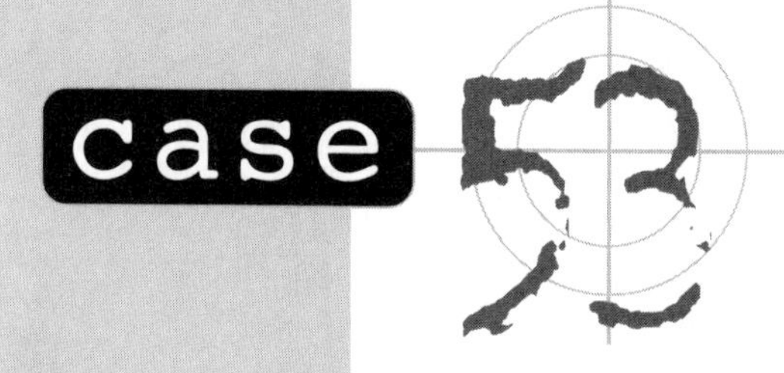

case 53

ID/CC A 5-year-old **girl** is brought to the pediatrician because her mother noticed **blood in her urine** and **diminished vision acuity.**

HPI Her family is **Mormon.** Her mother suffers from chronic renal failure.

PE VS: BP normal. PE: appears well nourished; bilateral **sensorineural hearing loss;** bilateral **cataracts.**

Labs CBC/PBS: normochromic, normocytic **anemia.** High-tone sensorineural loss detected on audiometry; elevated serum creatinine and BUN. UA: **proteinuria; hematuria;** RBC casts.

Gross Pathology Small, smooth kidneys.

Micro Pathology Longitudinal thinning and splitting of glomerular basement membrane, producing characteristic laminated appearance with glomerular sclerosis; interstitial infiltrate containing fat-filled macrophages (LARGE FOAM CELLS).

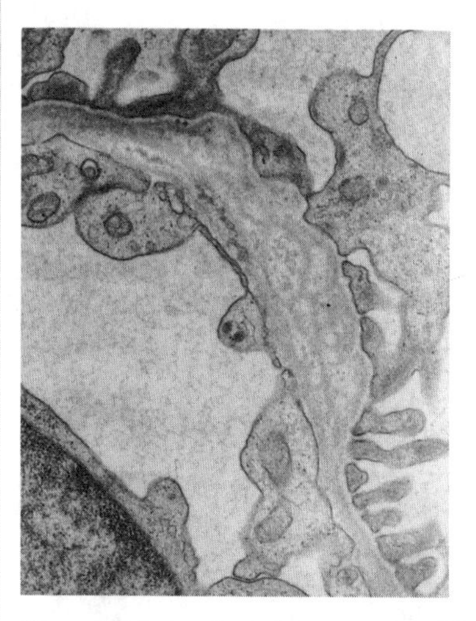

Figure 53-1. Laminated appearance of the glomerular basement membrane visible by electron microscopy.

case 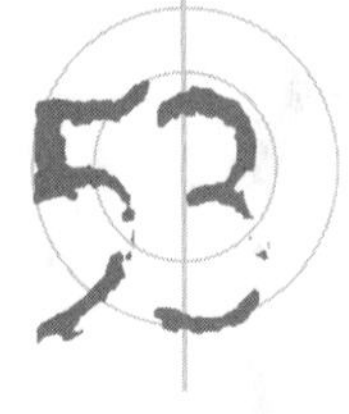

Alport Syndrome

Differential

Immunoglobulin A nephropathy
Thin membrane disease
Acute poststreptococcal glomerulonephritis
Urinary calculi
X-linked progressive hearing loss

Discussion

Alport syndrome can be autosomal dominant or x-linked and is caused by a defect in the α chain of type IV collagen. It is also called hereditary chronic nephritis and is progressive in males.

Treatment

ACE inhibitors; cyclosporine; renal transplantation.

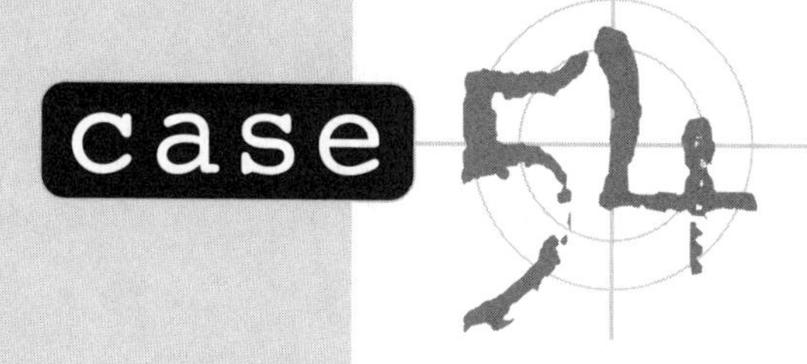

ID/CC A 45-year-old white woman complains of palpitations and shortness of breath, morning swelling of the eyes, arms, and legs, and numbness of the lower legs together with weight loss and fatigue.

HPI Her past medical history is unremarkable.

PE Mild cardiomegaly; **macroglossia;** pitting **edema** in lower extremities; **ascites; cardiac arrhythmia** on auscultation.

Labs UA: proteinuria. ECG: ventricular hypertrophy and low voltage **(restrictive cardiomyopathy).** Hypoproteinemia; hyperlipidemia.

Imaging CXR: massive cardiac enlargement. Echo: diastolic dysfunction; increased ventricular wall thickness; increased septal thickness; granular "sparkling" appearance.

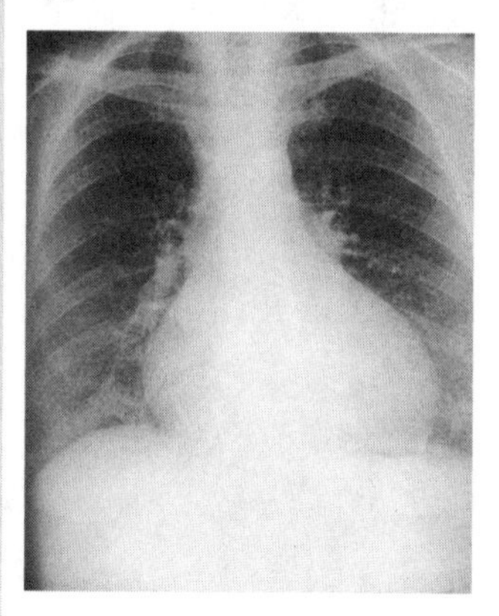

Figure 54-1. Chest radiograph showing massive cardiomegaly

Gross Pathology Pathologic deposition of amyloid glycoprotein in several organs, primarily heart, kidney, and rectal and gingival tissue.

Micro Pathology **Apple-green birefringence** in polarized light when stained **with Congo red.**

case 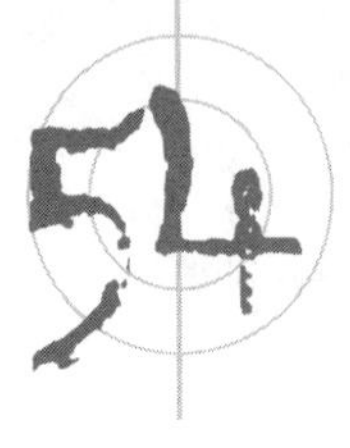

Amyloidosis—Primary

Differential

Multiple myeloma
Monoclonal gammopathy of uncertain origin
Familial renal amyloidosis
Dialysis-related amyloidosis
Transthyretin-related amyloidosis

Discussion

Primary amyloidosis commonly presents with nephrotic syndrome. Amyloidosis may be primary (in which the proteins are monoclonal **immunoglobulin light chain**) or secondary to chronic inflammatory states (especially rheumatoid arthritis and tuberculosis). The primary type is often associated with B-cell dyscrasias, especially **multiple myeloma**, and in these cases **Bence Jones proteins** are almost always present in the serum and urine.

Treatment

Supportive.

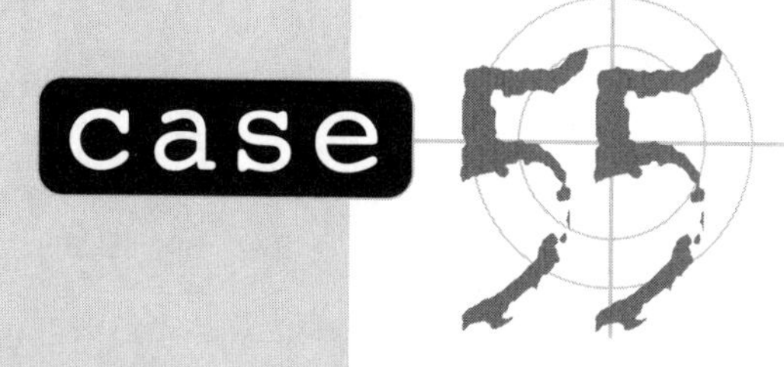

case 55

ID/CC A 56-year-old man complains of **urinary frequency** and interruption of the urinary stream over the past 6 months; he also complains of having to wake up multiple times during the night to urinate (NOCTURIA).

HPI The patient's history includes one episode of acute urinary retention 1 month ago that was relieved with catheterization. He denies any history of hematuria or back pain. He also admits to having a **reduced caliber of urine stream** and **terminal dribbling** as well as **urinary hesitancy.**

PE Digital rectal exam reveals **smooth enlargement of the prostate** protruding into the rectum; overlying rectal mucosa mobile; **bladder percussible up to umbilicus.**

Labs UA: 2+ bacteria; positive nitrite and leukocyte esterase. Prostate-specific antigen (PSA) levels normal; urodynamic studies demonstrate **bladder neck obstruction** with increased residual urine volume; mildly elevated serum creatinine and BUN.

Imaging US: benign-appearing enlargement of median lobe.

Gross Pathology Enlarged prostate with well-demarcated nodules up to 1 cm in diameter in **median lobe** of prostate.

Micro Pathology Both stroma and glands show **hyperplasia** on biopsy; fibromyoadenomatous hyperplasia seen in which proliferating glands are surrounded by proliferating smooth muscle cells and fibroblasts.

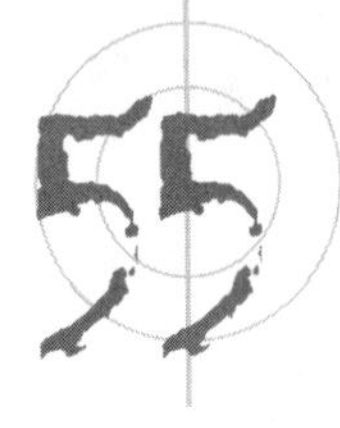

case 55

Benign Prostatic Hyperplasia

Differential

Prostatitis

Prostate cancer

Interstitial cystitis

Neurogenic bladder

Discussion

Age-dependent changes of estrogens and androgens are believed to cause benign prostatic hypertrophy (BPH); an increasing incidence is noted starting at 40 years of age. It affects up to 75% of men by the age of 80 years. It often arises in the periuretheral zone of the prostate, causing urinary symptoms. Complications include chronic hydronephrosis and pyleonephritis.

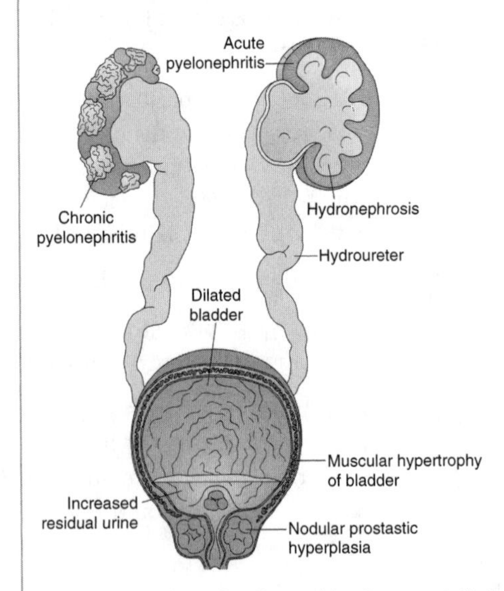

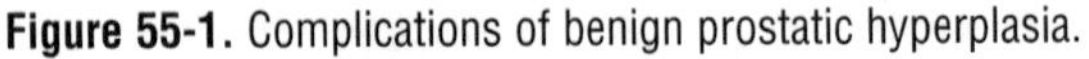
Figure 55-1. Complications of benign prostatic hyperplasia.

Treatment

Finasteride alleviates symptoms by inhibiting 5α-reductase, thereby blocking androgen action on prostate; tamsulosin relieves obstruction by blocking α_1 receptors in the prostate, bladder neck, and urethra; transurethral resection of prostate (TURP).

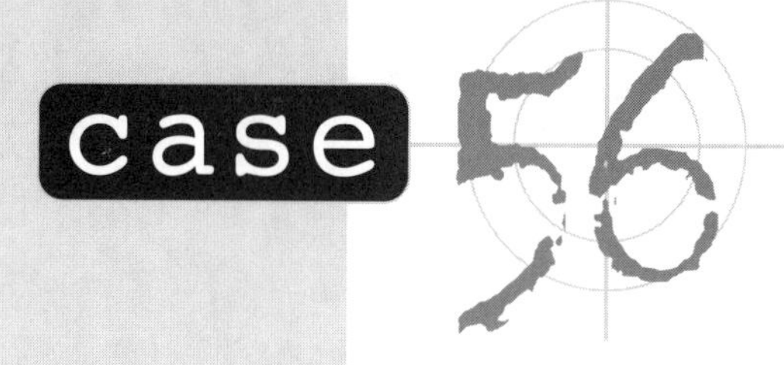

case 56

ID/CC A 65-year-old **white man** complains of **painless hematuria** of several-day duration.

HPI He is a **heavy smoker.**

PE Lungs clear; abdomen nontender; no palpable masses; genitalia within normal limits; no lymphadenopathy.

Labs CBC: slight normocytic, normochromic anemia. UA: **hematuria** and abundant epithelial cells.

Imaging IVP/Cystogram: **irregular filling defects** above trigone. MRI: Large mass within the bladder with involvement of lymph node.

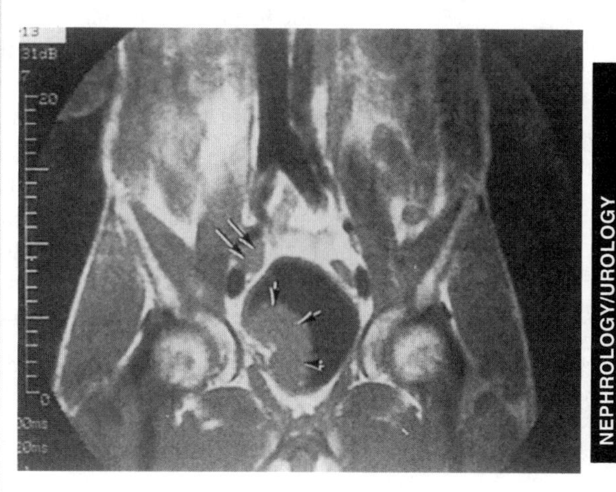

Figure 56-1. MRI scan of large muscle invasive bladder cancer (short arrows) and tumorous pelvic lymph node (long arrows).

Gross Pathology Nodular, **cauliflower-like** lesion with central necrosis and minimal invasion of bladder wall.

Micro Pathology Cytology of urine shows malignant cells. Biopsy of bladder shows grade I, stage B **transitional cell carcinoma** (TCC) arising from uroepithelium and projecting into bladder.

case 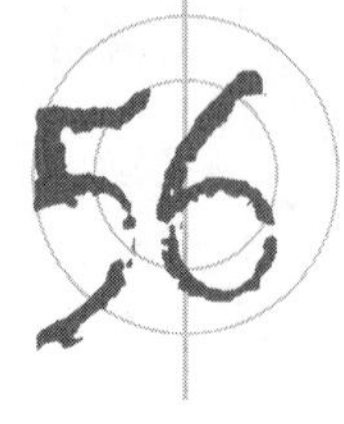

Bladder Cancer

Differential

Hemorrhagic cystitis
Nephrolithiasis
Renal cell carcinoma
Urethral trauma
Urinary tract infection

Discussion

There is a threefold increase in risk in men, and the average age at diagnosis is 65. Risk factors for papillary carcinoma of the bladder include industrial exposure to **arylamines** (especially 2-naphthylamine), **cigarette smoke, *Schistosoma haematobium*** infection (although most *Schistosoma* infections are associated with squamous neoplasia), **analgesic abuse** (especially phenacetin), and long-term **cyclophosphamide** therapy. Complications include invasion of perivesicular tissue, ureteral invasion with urinary obstruction (leading to hydronephrosis, pyelonephritis, and renal failure), and metastases to the lung, bone, and liver. TCC appears to be associated with mutations in the p53 tumor suppressor gene and deletions in chromosomes 9p and 9q.

Treatment

Surgery (cystoprostatectomy); radiotherapy; chemotherapy.

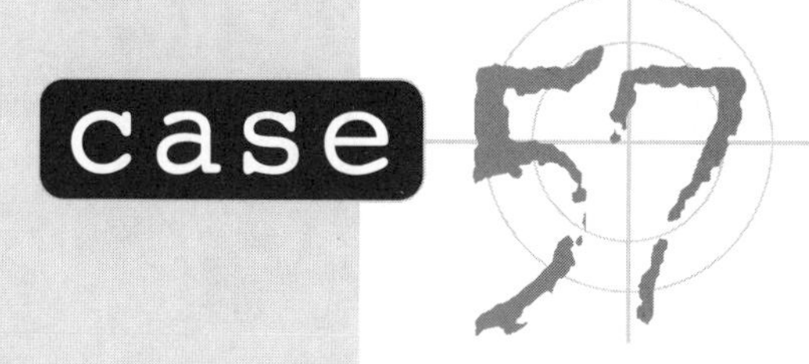

case 57

ID/CC A 65-year-old man presents with **acute urinary retention.**

HPI For the past few years, he has noted an **increased frequency** of micturition along with increased **hesitancy, urgency,** decreased force and stream of urine, and a feeling of **incomplete evacuation** of the bladder. For the past few months he has begun to experience **increasing fatigability and lassitude.**

PE Pallor; bladder full on abdominal examination; rectal exam reveals **grade III prostate enlargement.**

Labs CBC: normocytic anemia. Lytes: hypocalcemia; hyperphosphatemia. **Elevated BUN and creatinine.** UA: proteinuria; **no RBCs or casts seen.**

Imaging US, kidneys: **bilateral hydroureter and hydronephrosis.**

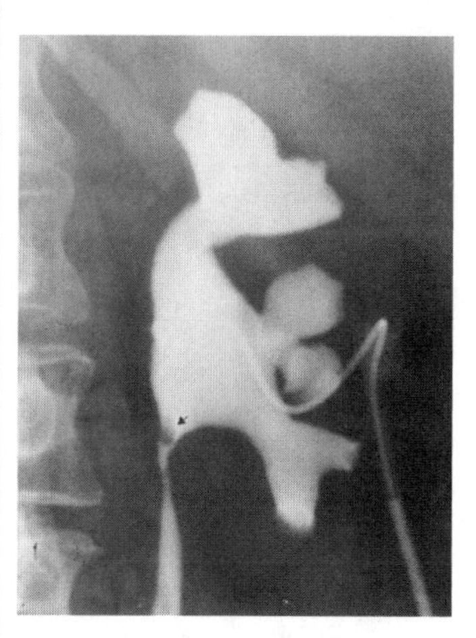

Figure 57-1. Hydronephrosis with dilation of the entire pelvocalyceal system.

Micro Pathology In addition to hydronephrosis and hydroureter, interstitial kidney disease is seen on microscopic examination.

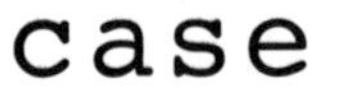

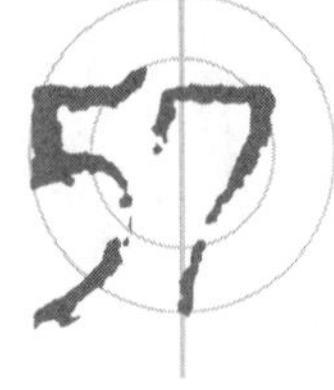

Bladder Outlet Obstruction

Differential

Benign prostatic hyperplasia
Bladder stone
Uterine fibroid (female)
Rectal cancer
Neurogenic bladder

Discussion

Obstructive nephropathy results from the **impaired outflow of urine** but may also **produce chronic interstitial damage.** Obstructive nephropathy is common in childhood (from congenital abnormalities) and in individuals older than 60 years, when benign prostatic hypertrophy and prostatic and gynecologic cancers become more common.

Treatment

Transurethral resection of the prostate (TURP) to relieve the obstruction is the basic and most useful step.

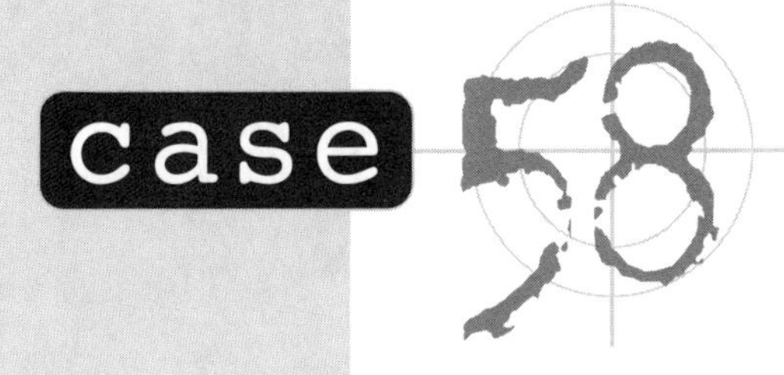

case 58

ID/CC A 48-year-old white woman is admitted to the hospital because of worsening **generalized edema** and weakness along with **hypertension.**

HPI She has a long history of type **I diabetes mellitus** but no history of hematuria, recent sore throat, or skin infections.

PE VS: **hypertension** (BP 160/110). PE: **generalized pitting edema;** no evidence of pleural effusion or ascites; lung bases clear on auscultation; JVP normal; neither kidney palpable; funduscopic exam reveals presence of **proliferative diabetic retinopathy.**

Labs **Elevated** fasting **blood sugar** (234 mg/dL); elevated glycosylated hemoglobin (10%); **elevated BUN and serum creatinine; decreased serum albumin; elevated blood cholesterol.** UA: presence of sugar and 3̣ **protein**; broad casts and **fatty casts;** elevated quantitative protein (3.5 g/24 hour).

Micro Pathology **Increased mesangial matrix** on renal biopsy; **thickening of capillary basement membrane** combined with acellular eosinophilic nodules in mesangium (KIMMELSTIEL–WILSON DISEASE); hyaline arteriosclerosis of both afferent and efferent arterioles; no immune complex deposits seen.

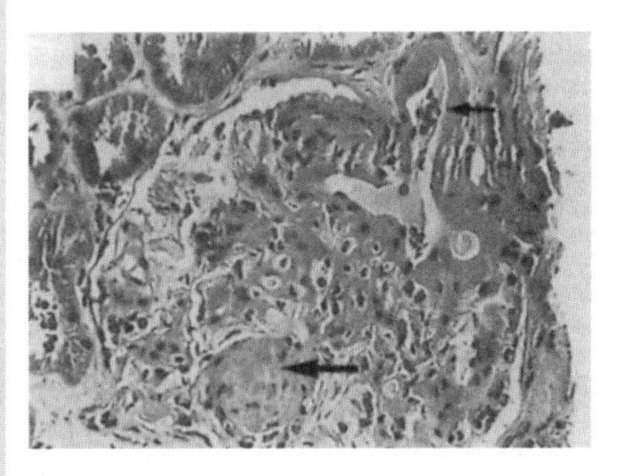

Figure 58-1. Increased mesangial matrix in the capillary loops (arrow).

NEPHROLOGY/UROLOGY

case 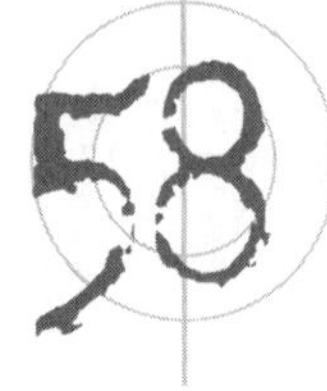

Diabetic Nephropathy

Differential

Myeloma kidney
Interstitial nephritis
Nephrosclerosis
Nephrotic syndrome

Discussion

Diabetic glomerulosclerosis is a renal manifestation of diabetic microangiopathy and presents at least 10 years after diabetes appears (more commonly in IDDM); it is usually the prelude to end-stage diabetic renal disease.

Treatment

Blood sugar control; ACE inhibitor or angiotensin receptor blocker to help prevent progression of diabetic nephropathy; control of systemic hypertension; dietary protein and phosphate restriction; avoidance of nephrotoxic drugs; dialysis or renal transplantation.

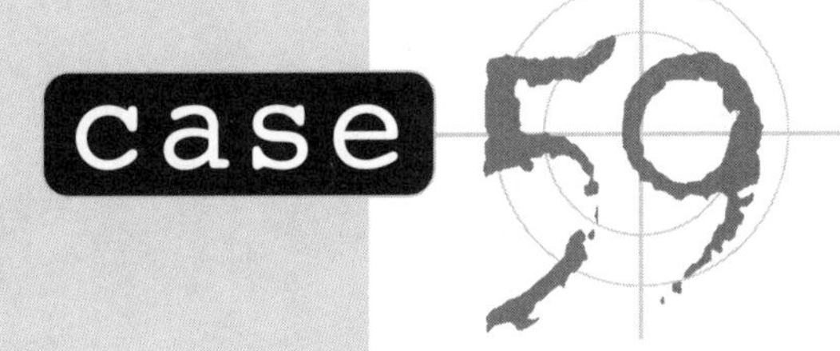

ID/CC A **25-year-old** white **man** complains of a chronic cough of several-month duration, accompanied by lightheadedness, fatigue, and malaise; yesterday he **coughed up blood.**

HPI He also describes intermittent fever and headaches in addition to small volumes of **dark orange urine.** He denies alcohol use but admits to being a heavy **smoker.**

PE Diffuse pulmonary crackles bilaterally.

Labs Azotemia. UA: oliguria; **hematuria;** proteinuria. **Antiglomerular basement membrane antibodies** in serum.

Imaging CXR: bilateral alveolar infiltrates.

Gross Pathology **Kidneys** enlarged and pale with decreased consistency.

Micro Pathology **Crescentic glomerulonephritis** with accumulation of neutrophils and macrophages in Bowman capsule; characteristic **linear IgG deposits in glomerular basement membrane and alveolar septa** on immunofluorescence; necrotizing hemorrhagic **alveolitis** on lung biopsy.

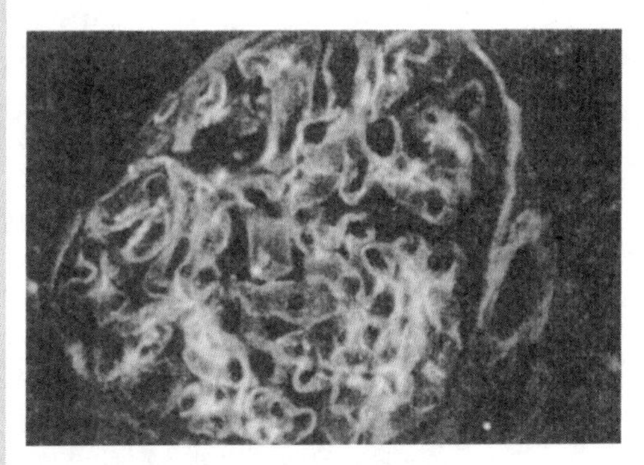

Figure 59-1. A continuous (linear) pattern of immunofluorescence staining for IgG is seen along glomerular capillary basement membranes and in Bowman capsule.

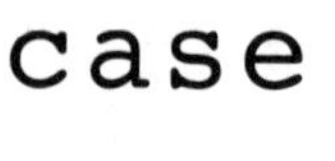
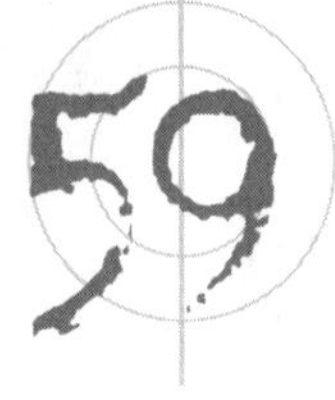

Goodpasture Syndrome

Differential

Poststreptococcal glomerulonephritis
Membranoproliferative glomerulonephritis
Rapidly progressive glomerulonephritis
Wegener granulomatosis

Discussion

Goodpasture syndrome is hemorrhagic alveolitis with nephritis and iron deficiency anemia caused by antiglomerular basement membrane antibodies (type II hypersensitivity reaction).

Treatment

Plasma exchange; corticosteroids; immunosuppressive therapy.

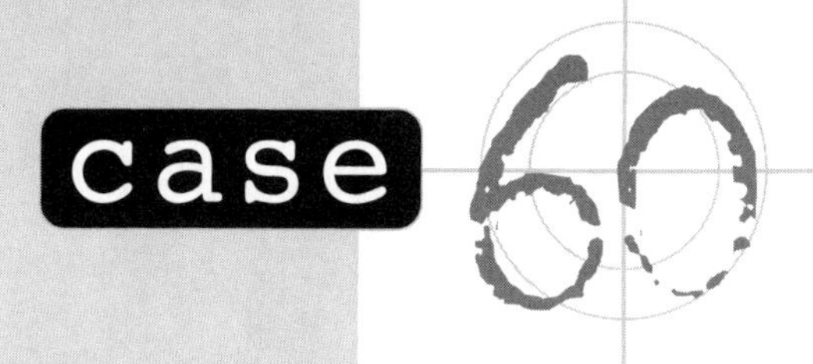

ID/CC A 45-year-old **black** man presents with uncontrolled **hypertension** and complains of severe occipital headache and ringing in his ears.

HPI He also reports **markedly diminished urine output over the past 24 hours.** On directed questioning, he also reports **some visual blurring.**

PE VS: **severe hypertension.** PE: funduscopy reveals presence of **papilledema** with **hypertensive retinopathy.**

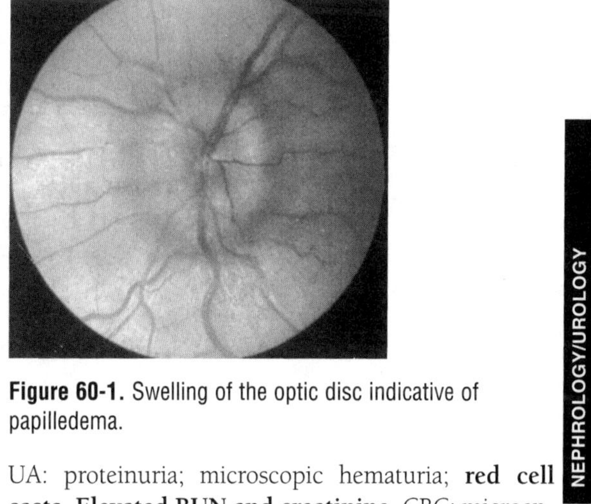

Figure 60-1. Swelling of the optic disc indicative of papilledema.

Labs UA: proteinuria; microscopic hematuria; **red cell casts. Elevated BUN and creatinine.** CBC: microangiopathic hemolytic anemia. ECG: left-axis deviation with left ventricular hypertrophy.

Imaging Echo: concentric left ventricular hypertrophy with reduced ejection fraction. US, abdomen: presence of **parenchymal renal disease in normal-sized kidneys.**

Micro Pathology Pathologic changes include **fibrinoid necrosis of arterioles** (NECROTIZING ARTERIOLITIS), **hyperplastic arteriolosclerosis** ("ONION SKINNING"), and necrotizing glomerulitis associated with a thrombotic microangiopathy.

case 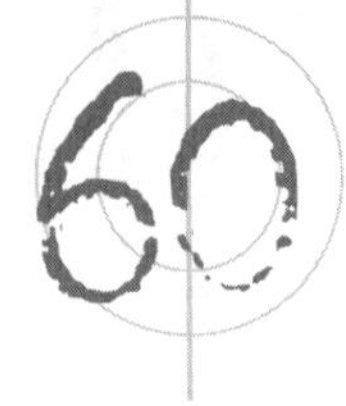

Hypertensive Renal Disease

Differential

Adrenal adenoma
Primary hyperaldosteronism
Hyperthyroidism
Renal artery stenosis

Discussion

Sodium nitroprusside is the safest and most effective drug for use in hypertensive emergencies; because it does not impair myocardial blood flow, it is especially useful in underlying ischemic heart disease. However, it is metabolized to cyanide and thiocyanate; therefore, prolonged use may lead to cyanide toxicity or to thiocyanate toxicity. Blood thiocyanate levels should be determined frequently.

Treatment

Reduction of diastolic blood pressure to at least 100 mmHg; maintain urine output >20 mL/hour. Multiple medications, including labetalol, hydralazine, nitroprusside, and enalaprilat, can be used to acutely lower blood pressure.

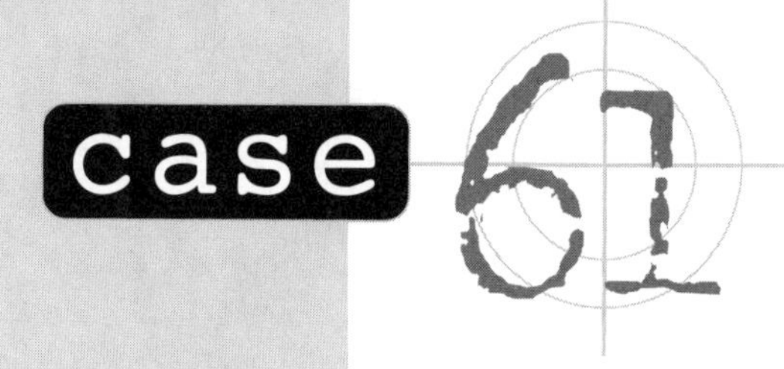

ID/CC	A 22-year-old white man complains of recurrent episodes of "**bloody urine**" that lasted for several days **in conjunction** with a **URI.**
HPI	He was well until the onset of symptoms.
PE	Pallor; slight palpebral edema.
Labs	UA: proteinuria; **red cell casts in urine**; gross hematuria. **Increased serum IgA.**
Micro Pathology	Focal glomerulonephritis involving only selected glomeruli with **mesangial proliferation** and segmental necrosis with crescents; immunofluorescence typically reveals mesangial **IgA deposits** with some IgM, IgG, and C3.

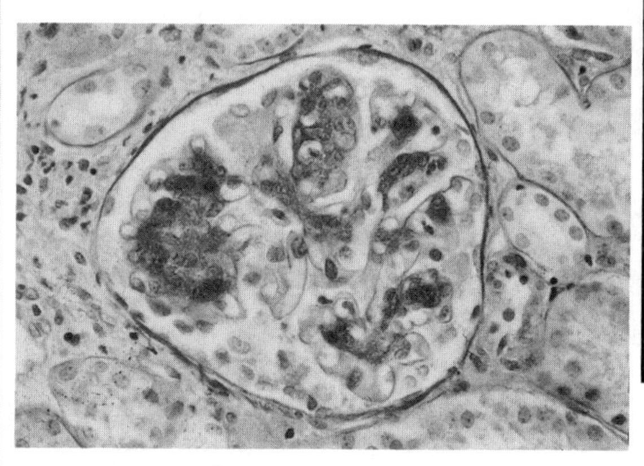

Figure 61-1. Segmental mesangial hypercellularity and matrix expansion due to mesangial immune deposits.

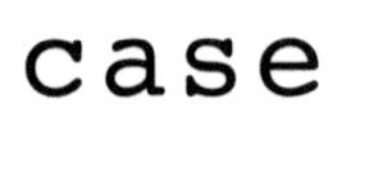

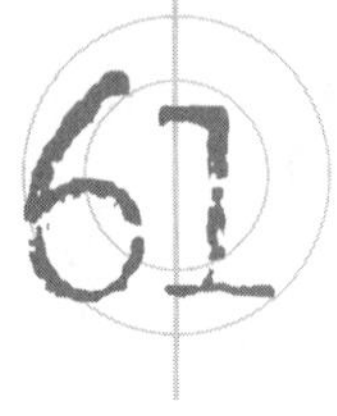

IgA Nephropathy

Differential

Alport syndrome
Crescentic glomerulonephritis
Membranoproliferative glomerulonephritis
Poststreptococcal glomerulonephritis
Lupus nephritis

Discussion

IgA nephropathy is idiopathic but associated with upper respiratory or GI infections lacking a latency period (vs. poststreptococcal glomerulonephritis). Lesions are variable and may be mesangioproliferative, focal proliferative, or possibly crescentic glomerulonephritis. The glomerular pathology seen in Berger disease is similar to that seen in **Henoch–Schönlein purpura,** which is seen in children. It is seen with increased frequency in patients with celiac disease and liver disease (due to defective IgA clearance). **Chronic renal failure may ultimately develop.**

Treatment

Supportive; ACE inhibitors for hypertension and proteinuria; fish oil; immunosuppressive therapy in selected cases; IgA deposits commonly reappear following kidney transplantation.

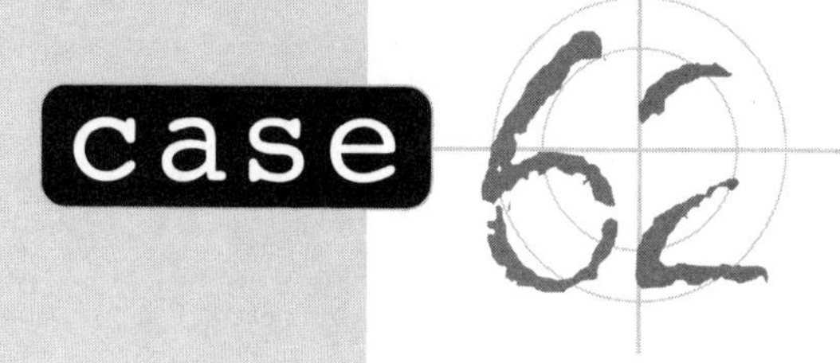

ID/CC A **30-year-old black woman** presents with **pain** in both her knee **joints** and in the small joints of the hand together with mild fever, anorexia, weight loss, and loss of hair.

HPI She also has a history of **recurrent oral ulcerations** and a **photosensitive skin rash.** No joint deformities are reported.

PE VS: hypertension. PE: oral **aphthous ulcers** noted; erythematous **photosensitive skin rash**; "**butterfly rash**" over malar area of face; pallor; no abdominal or renal bruits heard.

Labs CBC: normocytic, normochromic **anemia.** UA: microscopic hematuria with **RBC casts** in addition to proteinuria. **Elevated BUN and creatinine; antinuclear antibodies positive** in high titer; **LE cell phenomenon** positive; **anti-Sm antibody and anti-ds DNA antibody positive; VDRL positive** but FTA-ABS negative; low serum complement levels.

Micro Pathology Renal biopsy reveals features of **diffuse proliferative glomerulonephritis.** Electron microscopy reveals **immune complex deposits** that are typically **subendothelial** and form "**wire loops.**"

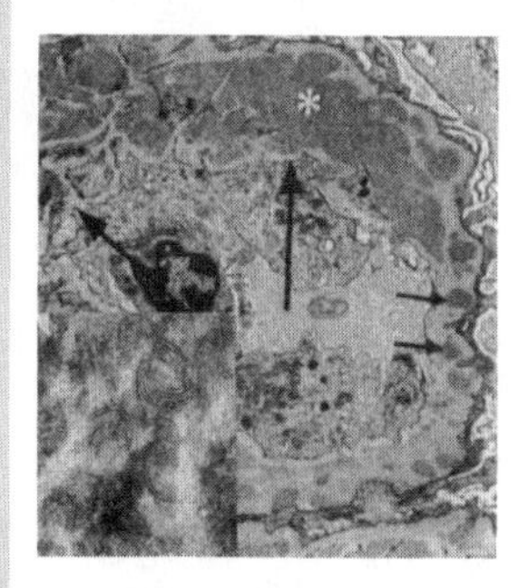

Figure 62-1. The electron micrograph reveals large subendothelial (asterisk) and intramembranous (short arrows) deposits with mesangial interposition (long arrow).

NEPHROLOGY/UROLOGY

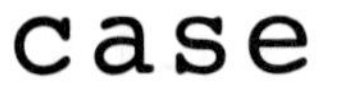

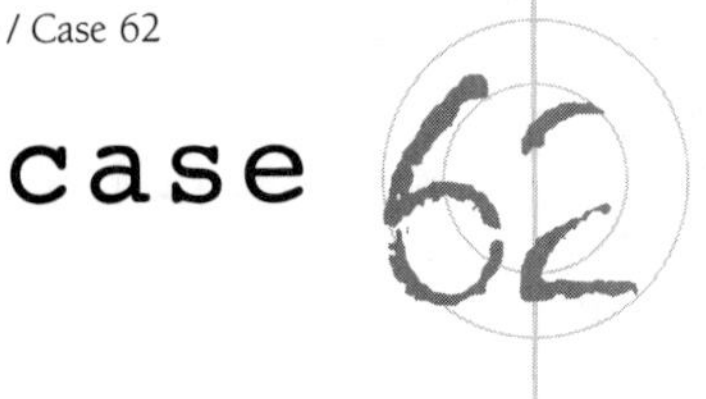

Lupus Nephritis

Differential

Diffuse proliferative glomerulonephritis
Membranous glomerulonephritis
Polyarteritis nodosa
Wegener granulomatosis

Discussion

There are five patterns of lupus nephritis. Class I is normal by light, EM, and immunofluorescence microscopy. Class II presents as **mesangial lupus glomerulonephritis** and is found in about 25% of patients; it is associated with minimal hematuria or proteinuria. Class III is characterized by **focal proliferative** glomerulonephritis and is associated with recurrent hematuria and mild renal insufficiency. Class IV is described in this case and is by far the most common form. Class V presents as **membranous glomerulonephritis** and is seen in 15% of cases; it induces severe proteinuria or nephrotic syndrome.

Treatment

Corticosteroids; cytotoxic drugs (cyclophosphamide, azathioprine, and chlorambucil); long-term hemodialysis or transplant.

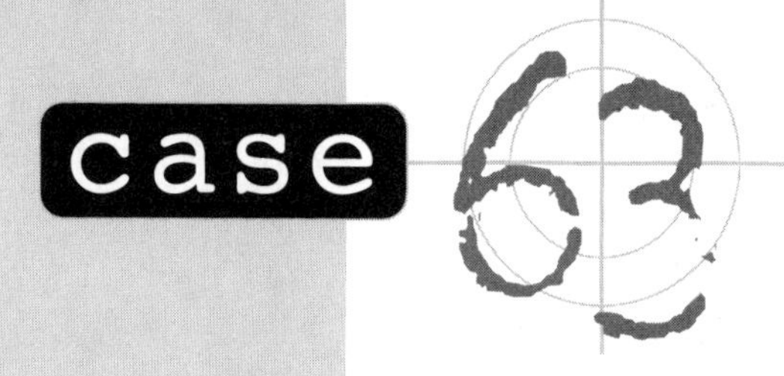

case 63

ID/CC An 11-year-old white girl is brought to the pediatrician because of headache, chest palpitations, and ringing in her ears together with **generalized edema.**

HPI She has no history of dyspnea, sore throat, skin infections, or fever. Careful questioning reveals that she has also had **hematuria.**

PE VS: hypertension (BP 140/100). PE: **generalized** (including periorbital) **pitting edema;** JVP normal; lung bases clear; neither kidney palpable; no evidence of pleural effusion or ascites.

Labs Elevated BUN and serum creatinine; decreased serum albumin; elevated serum triglycerides; serum **hypocomplementemia;** antinuclear antibody (ANA) negative; normal ASO titers. UA: **fatty casts and oval bodies in addition to proteins.**

Micro Pathology Diffuse glomerular involvement with thickened capillary walls and lobular mesangial proliferation on light microscopy. **Splitting of basement membrane causing railroad-track "TRAM TRACK" appearance** with PAS reagent or silver stain.

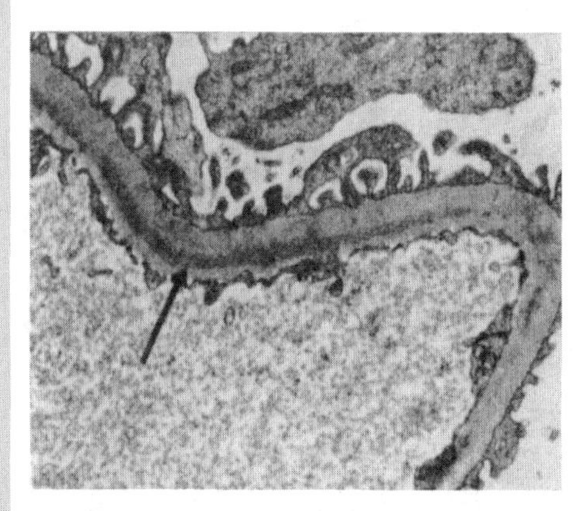

Figure 63-1. Electron micrograph of an intramembranous dense deposit (arrow).

case 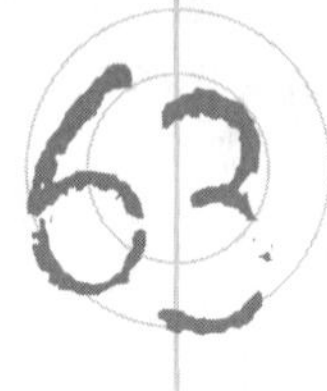

Membranoproliferative Glomerulonephritis

Differential

Poststreptococcal glomerulonephritis
Rapidly progressive glomerulonephritis
Lupus nephritis
IgA nephropathy

Discussion

Membranoproliferative glomerulonephritis (MPGN) is idiopathic but may be associated with inherited deficiencies of complement components and partial lipodystrophy. It is subdivided into two types: type I MPGN (both classic and alternative complement pathways activated) and type II MPGN (dense deposit disease; activation of alternate complement pathway). The majority of patients with MPGN will go on to develop **chronic renal failure.** There is a **high recurrence rate** following renal transplantation.

Treatment

Corticosteroids; renal transplantation.

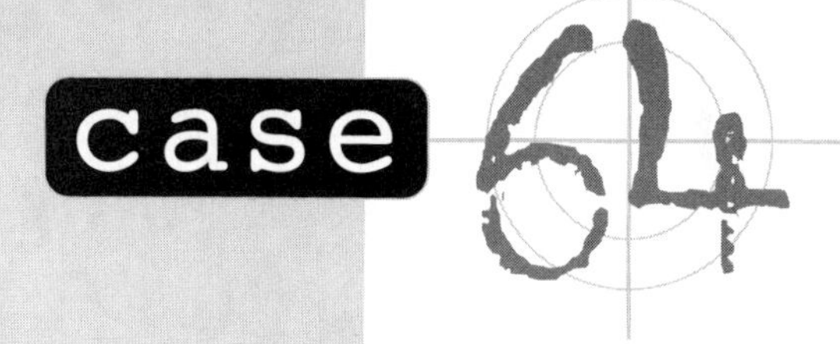

case 64

ID/CC A 47-year-old black woman with diabetes complains of weight loss, progressive shortness of breath, and **swelling of the lower legs** and arms.

HPI Her past medical history is unremarkable.

PE Pallor; pitting edema in extremities; decreased lung sounds with crackles bilaterally in lower lung fields; **periorbital edema; ascites.**

Labs UA: **proteinuria** (>3.5 g/24 hour); lipiduria with oval fat bodies and fatty and waxy casts in urinary sediment. **Hypoalbuminemia (<3 g/dl); hyperlipidemia** (serum cholesterol 250 mg/dL).

Gross Pathology Kidneys enlarged, pale, and rubbery; renal vein thrombosis may be present.

Micro Pathology **Thickened basement membrane;** subepithelial deposits of IgG and C3 along basement membrane seen in "**spike and dome**" pattern on methenamine silver stain; immune deposits in a "**lumpy-bumpy**" (discontinuous) pattern on immunofluorescence.

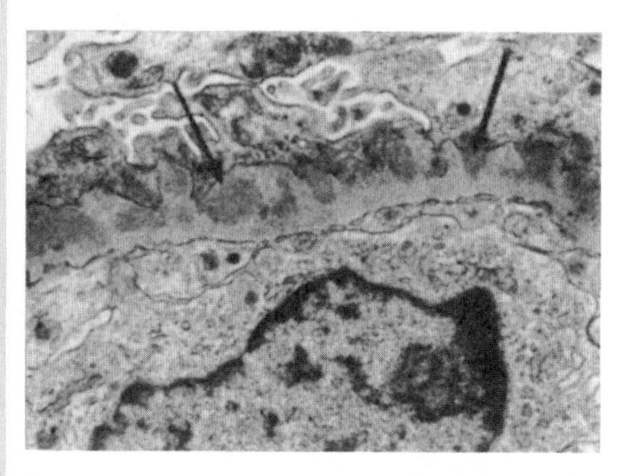

Figure 64-1. Subepithelial deposits of IgG and C3 along basement membrane seen by electron microscopy.

case 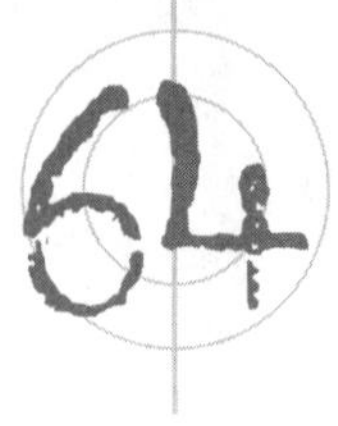

Membranous Glomerulonephritis

Differential

Focal segmental glomerulonephritis
Membranoproliferative glomerulonephritis
Minimal change disease
Myocardial infarction
Congestive heart failure

Discussion

Nephrotic syndrome may be idiopathic or caused by membranous glomerulonephritis (the most common cause in adults), minimal change disease (LIPOID NEPHROSIS) (the most common in children), focal glomerulosclerosis, or membranoproliferative glomerulonephritis. Patients with nephrotic syndrome have **hypercoagulability** secondary to loss of antithrombin III in the urine (e.g., increased incidence of peripheral vein thrombosis).

Treatment

Corticosteroids; cyclophosphamide; renal transplantation; ACE inhibitors reduce urinary protein loss.

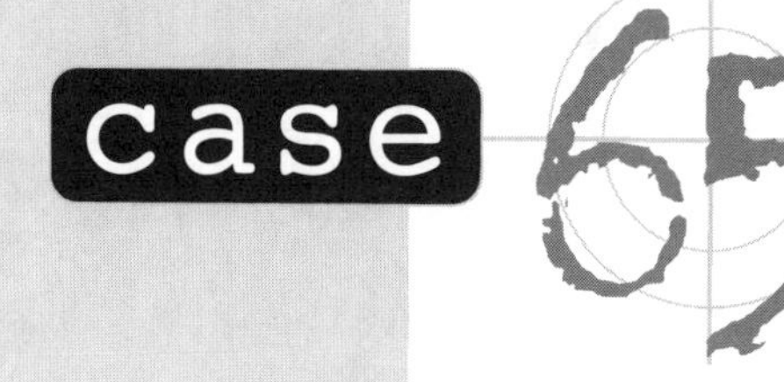

ID/CC A **5-year-old** caucasian girl presents with **generalized edema** and abdominal distention, producing respiratory embarrassment.

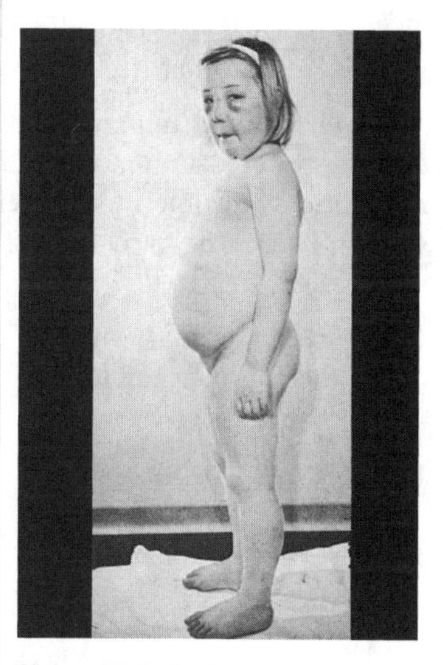

Figure 65-1. Periorbital edema, abdominal distension, and bilateral lower extremity edema (anasarca).

HPI The child had a **URI** 1 week ago.

PE VS: BP normal. PE: generalized pitting edema; free **ascitic fluid** in peritoneal cavity; shifting dullness and fluid thrill present; normal funduscopic exam.

Labs UA: 4**proteinuria** (>3 g/24 hour). **Hypoalbuminemia; hypercholesterolemia;** hypertriglyceridemia; decreased serum ionic calcium; normal C3 levels; normal serum creatinine and BUN.

Gross Pathology Kidneys slightly enlarged, soft, and yellowish.

Micro Pathology Light microscopy and immunofluorescent studies **normal on renal biopsy** (no evidence of immune complex deposition). EM reveals uniform and diffuse loss of the podocytic foot processes.

case 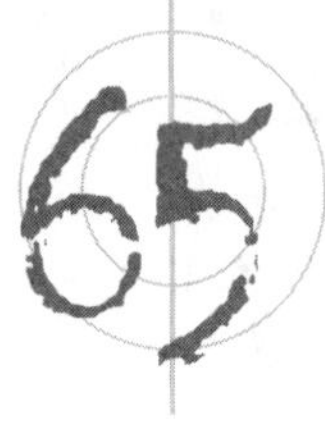

Minimal Change Disease

Differential

Heart failure

Membranoproliferative glomerulonephritis

Membranous glomerulonephritis

Focal segmental glomerulonephritis

Discussion

Also called **lipoid nephrosis,** minimal change disease is the most common cause of idiopathic **nephrotic syndrome in children** and is associated with infections or vaccinations. It carries a **good prognosis.**

Treatment

Corticosteroids; salt-restricted diet; diuretics; electrolyte therapy and monitoring.

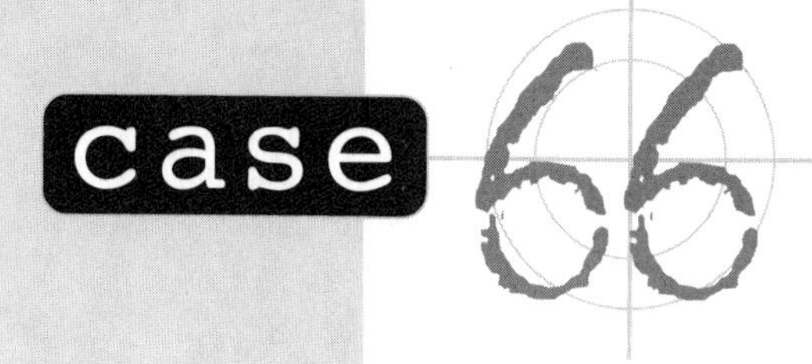

case 66

ID/CC A 68-year-old **black** man complains of **dysuria, progressively increased urinary frequency**, and **back pain** that has lasted several months.

HPI He reports **high animal-fat intake.**

PE Nodular, **rock-hard, irregular area of induration** in **peripheral lobe** of prostate on digital rectal exam; **midline furrow** between prostatic lobes **obscured; extension to seminal vesicles** detected.

Labs **Markedly elevated prostate-specific antigen** (PSA) and **acid phosphatase.**

Imaging Transrectal US, prostate: **hypoechoic masses** in peripheral zone with extension to seminal vesicles. Nuc, bone scan: **hot lesions of spine, sacrum, and pelvic bones** (axial skeleton). CT/MR: prostate mass with capsular penetration and enlarged seminal vesicles.

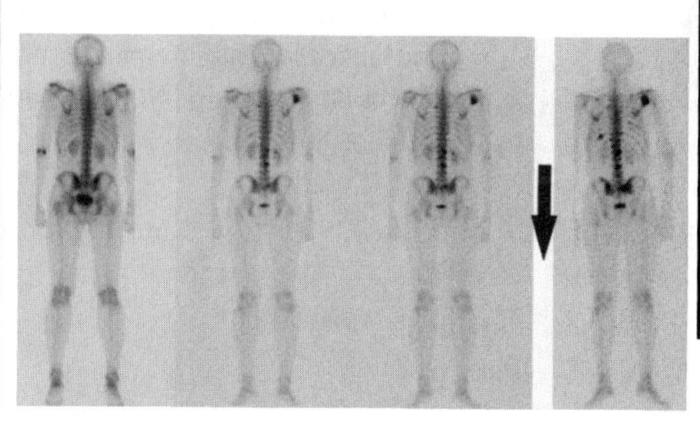

Figure 66-1. Technetium 99m bone scan in a patient with lesions of the **spine, sacrum, and pelvic bones.**

Gross Pathology Irregularly enlarged, firm, nodular prostate.

Micro Pathology Core needle biopsy of prostate reveals single layer of malignant neoplastic cells arranged haphazardly in adenoplastic stroma.

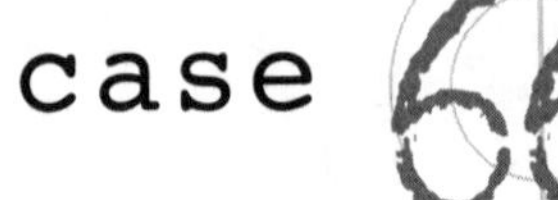
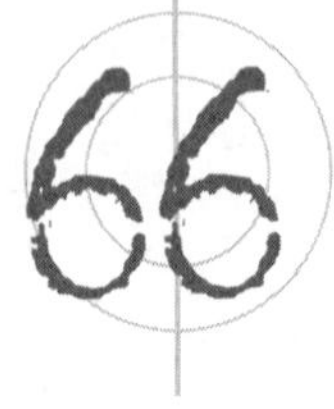

Prostate Carcinoma

Differential

Prostatitis

Benign prostatic hyperplasia

Multiple myeloma

Urinary tract infection

Discussion

A primary malignant neoplasm of the prostate commonly arising from the peripheral zone (70%), prostate carcinoma is the **most common male cancer.** Its prognosis and treatment depend heavily on stage. Most cases are diagnosed in **asymptomatic** men on digital rectal exam. Prostate cancer exhibits **hematogenous dissemination**, most commonly to **bone**, forming **osteoblastic lesions.** The tumor can also invade sacral nerve roots, causing significant pain.

Treatment

Prostatectomy or radiation for early stage (disease confined to the prostate); radiation alone for locally advanced disease or palliative radiation with bone metastasis: orchiectomy; leuprolide; antiandrogens such as flutamide.

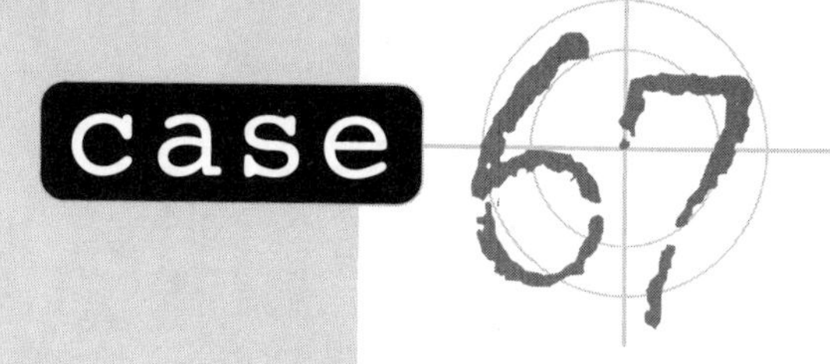

case 67

ID/CC	A 60-year-old white man complains of right **flank pain** and **hematuria.**
HPI	He has been a **heavy smoker** for the past 24 years; he **lost 5 pounds over the past month** and is not on a diet.
PE	VS: low-grade fever; moderate hypertension. PE: pallor; **palpable mass** in right flank.
Labs	Elevated ESR. CBC/PBS: normocytic, normochromic **anemia**. UA: gross **hematuria.**
Imaging	IVP/CT/US: mass in upper pole of right kidney. MR: no invasion of renal vein or inferior vena cava (IVC).
Gross Pathology	Yellowish areas of necrotic tissue with focal areas of hemorrhage within renal parenchyma.
Micro Pathology	Polygonal **clear cells** (containing glycogen) with evidence of cytologic atypia invading renal parenchyma.

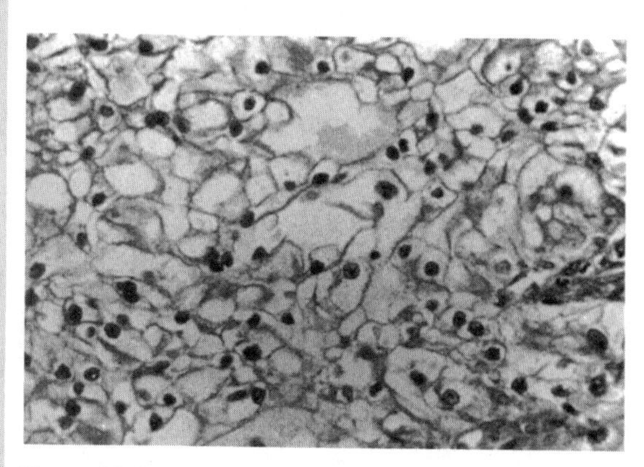

Figure 67-1. Polygonal **clear cells.**

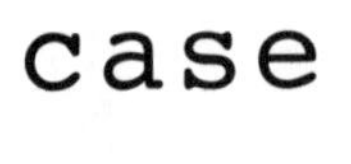

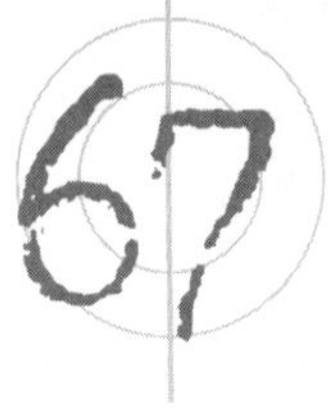

Renal Cell Carcinoma

Differential

Non-Hodgkin lymphoma
Chronic pyelonephritis
Wilms tumor
Renal cyst
Angiomyolipoma

Discussion

The **most common renal tumor**, renal cell carcinoma is frequently sporadic but is seen in association with **von Hippel–Lindau syndrome** and dialysis-related **acquired polycystic kidney disease.** It frequently invades the **renal vein and IVC** and metastasizes to lungs and bone via hematogenous dissemination. It can also cause **paraneoplastic syndromes** (secondary to the production of erythropoietin, parathyroid-like hormone, ACTH, and renin).

Treatment

Right **nephrectomy;** consider renal-sparing partial nephrectomy; chemotherapy, immunotherapy, and radiation treatment may be considered for advanced or metastatic disease.

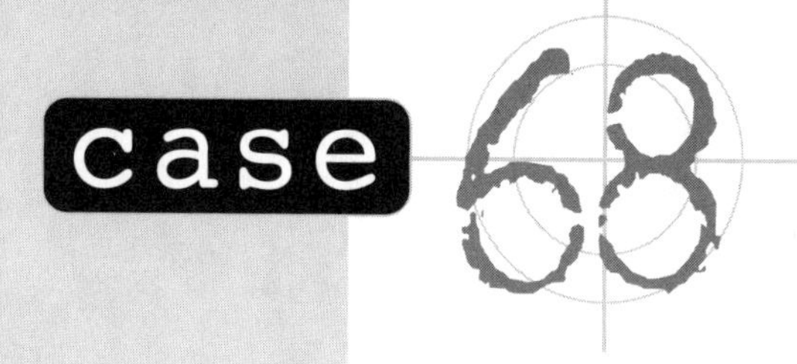

case 68

ID/CC A 63-year-old white man complains of **sudden-onset pain** in the right **flank** together with gross **hematuria,** nausea, and vomiting.

HPI He is **overweight,** has been diabetic for 15 years, is a heavy **smoker** and drinker, and has been surgically treated for **aortofemoral occlusive disease** (graft).

PE VS: no fever; mild hypertension (BP 150/100). PE: **acute distress;** pallor; sweating; severe right flank pain; **xanthelasma** in both eyelids.

Labs Normal BUN and creatinine. UA: **hematuria.** ECG: old silent anterior wall myocardial infarction. Elevated **LDH.**

Imaging CT, abdomen: **wedge-shaped, nonenhancing lesions in right kidney.** US, renal: edematous kidney with focal region of decreased color flow.

NEPHROLOGY/UROLOGY

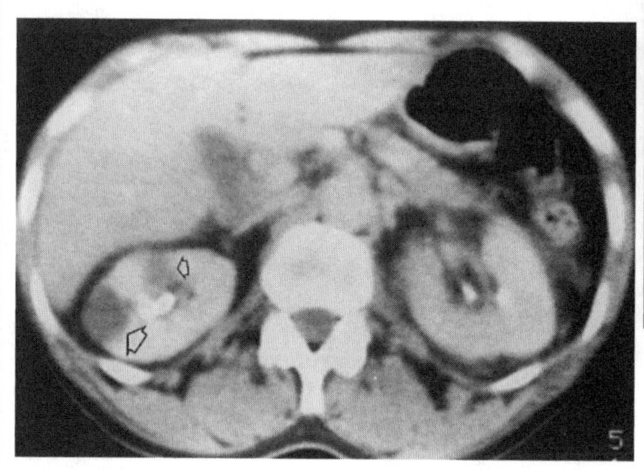

Figure 68-1. Wedge-shaped, nonenhancing lesions in right kidney.

Gross Pathology Pale, yellowish white, wedge-shaped area with hemorrhagic necrosis in renal cortex.

Micro Pathology Coagulation necrosis involving renal cortical nephrons extending into corticomedullary junction.

case 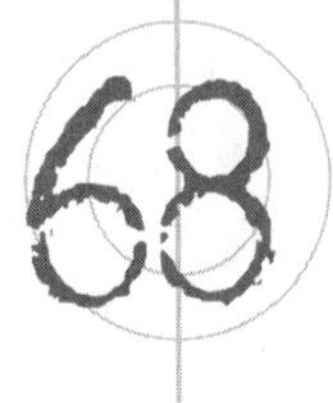

Renal Infarction

Differential

Cystitis
Glomerulonephritis
Nephrolithiasis
Renal cell carcinoma

Discussion

Risk factors for embolic events include **atherosclerosis** and mural thrombi in the heart and aorta, infectious endocarditis vegetations, and atheromatous plaques in the aorta. Complications from renal artery embolism include renal failure, hypertension, acute pyelonephritis, and renal abscess.

Treatment

Remove arterial obstruction by thrombolysis; heparin anticoagulation to prevent recurrence.

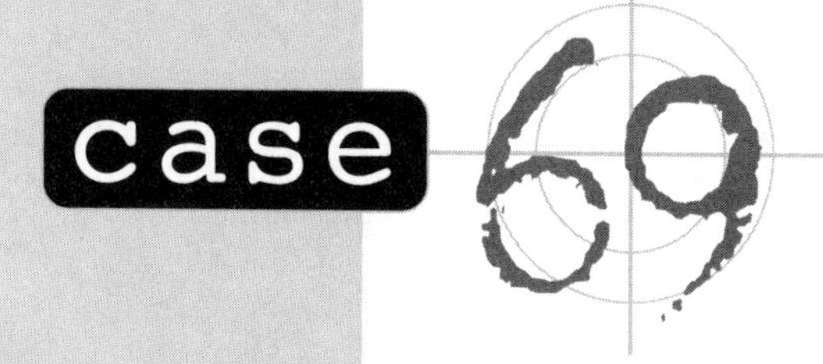

case 69

ID/CC A **30-year-old** white woman is found to be **hypertensive** on routine physical exam.

HPI She claims to have **no history of hypertension** and denies any changes in lifestyle or excessive stress.

PE VS: **hypertension** (BP 175/105). PE: loud S2; funduscopic exam normal; **abdominal bruit** present.

Labs **Elevated plasma renin;** hypokalemia.

Imaging Angio, renal: confirmatory; bilateral **renal artery stenosis in a "string of pearls" pattern.**

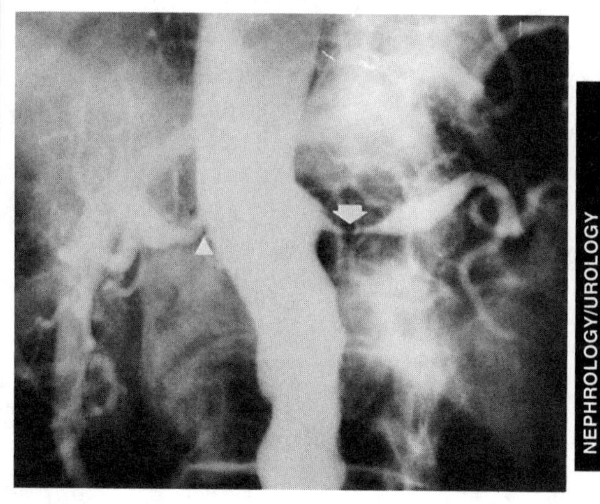

Figure 69-1. Bilateral "string of pearls" pattern of the renal artery.

Gross Pathology In fibromuscular dysplasia, the renal artery lumen is decreased due to hyperplastic fibrotic wall thickening.

Micro Pathology Muscular hyperplasia with fibrosis and segmental stenosis.

case 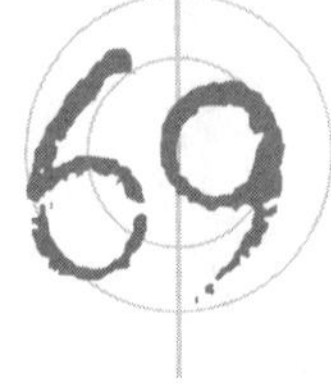

Renovascular Hypertension

Differential

Essential hypertension
Atherosclerosis
Nephrosclerosis
Acute renal failure

Discussion

Renovascular hypertension is secondary systemic hypertension caused by hypersecretion of renin from hypoperfused kidney(s). It is most often caused by **fibromuscular dysplasia (young white women)** or **atherosclerosis (older men)** and accounts for <5% of all causes of hypertension.

Treatment

ACE inhibitors (contraindicated in bilateral renal artery stenosis); calcium channel blockers; balloon angioplasty; stenting; surgical correction.

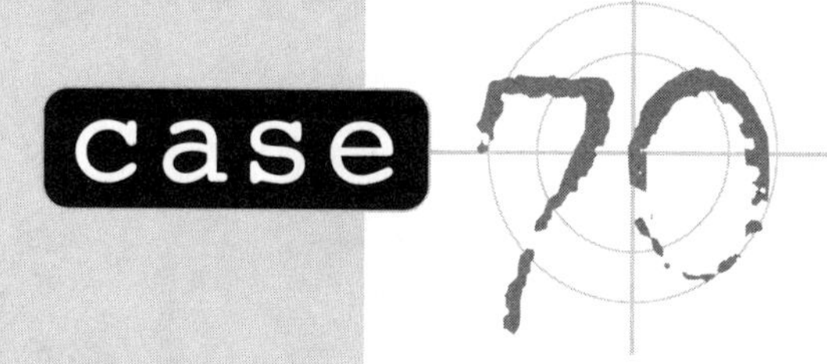

case 70

ID/CC A **36-year-old** white man presents with **progressive painless enlargement of the left testicle** of 2-month duration.

HPI He also complains of a sense of heaviness in his scrotum. He denies any history of pain or trauma at the site.

PE Walnut-sized, nontender, smooth, **firm mass at upper end of left testicle; mass does not transilluminate;** epididymis and vas deferens normal on palpation; prostate and seminal vesicles normal on digital rectal exam; abdominal lymph nodes not palpable; no hepatomegaly.

Labs Normal levels of hCG; **normal levels of serum α-fetoprotein and LDH; histologic** diagnosis based on postoperative specimen study.

Imaging CXR: no metastasis. US, abdomen and pelvis/scrotum: solid intratesticular mass. CT, abdomen and pelvis: no metastasis.

Gross Pathology Solid white bulging mass within testis.

Micro Pathology Sheets of germ cells containing clear cytoplasm with lymphocytes in fibrous stroma.

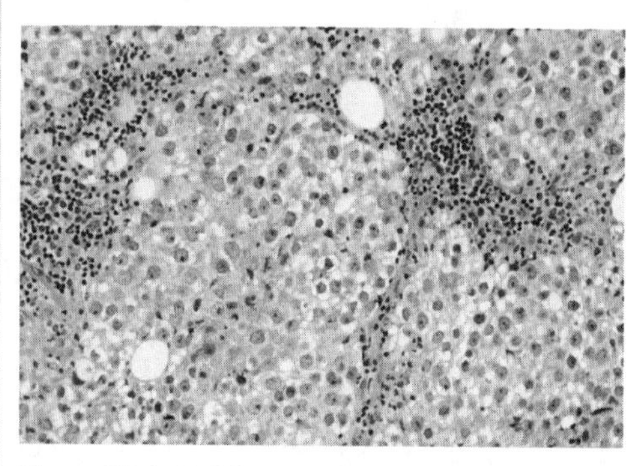

Figure 70-1. Solid nests of germ cells surrounded by fibrous stoma containing lymphocytes.

case 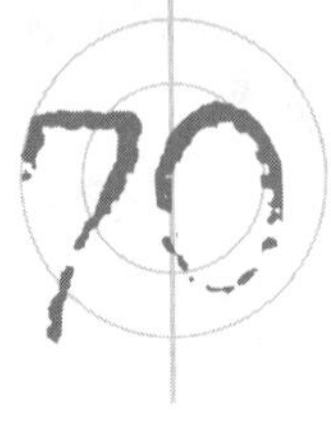

Seminoma

Differential

Epididymitis
Hydrocele
Testicular choriocarcinoma
Nonseminomatous testicular tumor
Testicular teratocarcinoma

Discussion

Seminoma is the most common type of germ cell tumor. Dysgerminomas in ovaries are histologically similar. Tumors are extremely **radiosensitive** and are associated with a good prognosis. **Cryptorchidism** predisposes to the development of testicular tumors.

Treatment

Orchiectomy followed by retroperitoneal lymph node dissection; chemotherapy with cisplatin; radiotherapy.

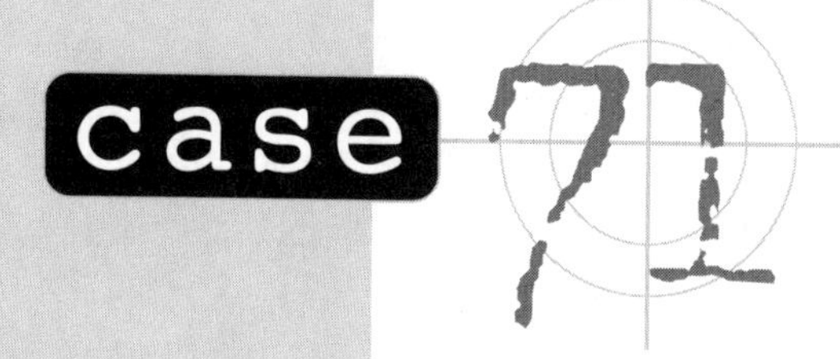

case 71

ID/CC A 30-year-old man complains of a small **painless nodular swelling over his right testicle** that he noticed a few months ago, coupled with **increasing growth of his breast tissue.**

HPI He also complains of mild shortness of breath on exertion (DYSPNEA), cough, and blood-streaked sputum.

PE VS: normal. PE: bilateral gynecomastia (breast tissue palpable); small, **pea-shaped swelling** involving the **right testicle;** testicular sensation lost; no transillumination; **left supraclavicular lymphadenopathy;** hepatomegaly.

Labs CBC: mild anemia. Serum **β-hCG elevated.**

Imaging CXR: two "cannonball" parenchymal masses (due to metastases). CT, abdomen: enlarged retroperitoneal lymph nodes and multiple hepatic metastases. US, scrotum: complex, solid right testicular mass.

Gross Pathology Small, pea-shaped hemorrhagic mass seen in right testicle.

Micro Pathology Polygonal, comparatively uniform **cytotrophoblastic cells** with clear cytoplasm growing in sheets and cords, mixed with **multinucleate syncytiotrophoblastic cells** that have **eosinophilic vacuolated cytoplasm** with readily **demonstrable hCG;** no well-developed villi seen.

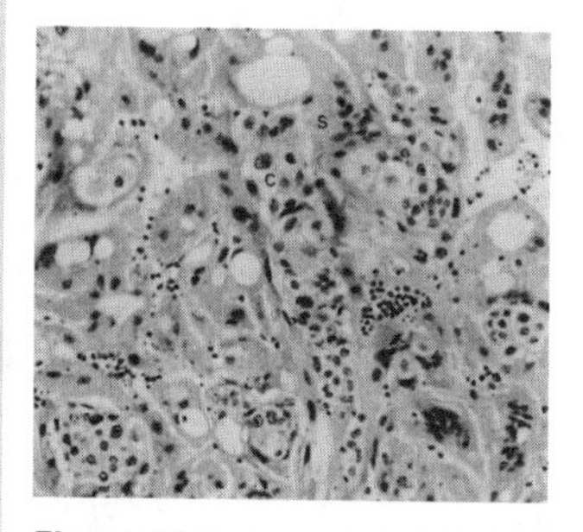

Figure 71-1. Irregularly interlacing aggregates of syncytiotrophoblast (S) and cytotrophoblast (C) without villi.

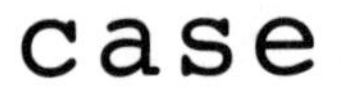
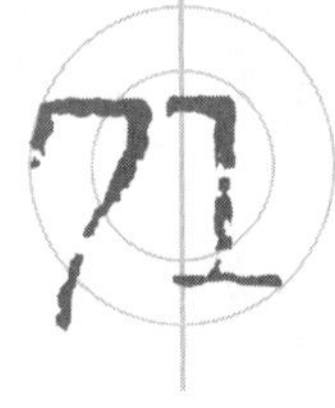

Testicular Choriocarcinoma

Differential

Epididymitis
Hydrocele
Testicular seminoma
Nonseminomatous testicular tumor
Testicular teratocarcinoma
Non-Hodgkin lymphoma

Discussion

Choriocarcinoma is the **most malignant** of all testicular tumors; it metastasizes relatively early via both the **lymphatics** and the **bloodstream** even when it remains very small locally. **Follow-up with β-hCG levels.**

Treatment

Chemotherapy with **cisplatin, etoposide, and bleomycin** in some combination, followed by **radical inguinal orchiectomy** and **retroperitoneal lymph node dissection**; gynecomastia regresses once the source of hCG (the tumor) is removed.

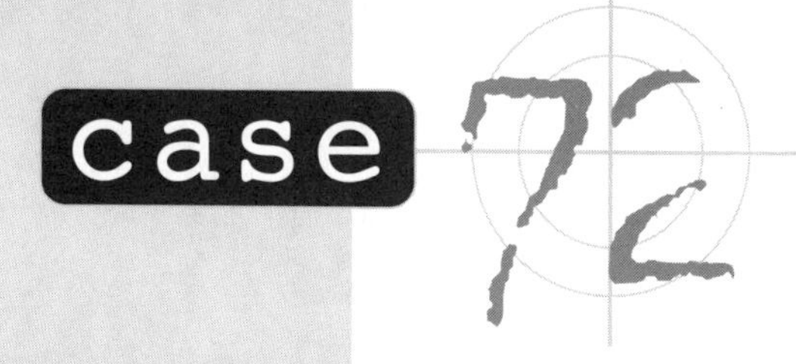

case 72

ID/CC A newborn baby is evaluated for **ambiguous external genitalia.**

HPI The baby was delivered vaginally at full term without any pre-, intra-, or postnatal complications; the mother did not take **hormones** or any other **drugs during pregnancy.**

PE **Incompletely virilized external genitalia;** hypospadias; **bilateral inguinal swelling.**

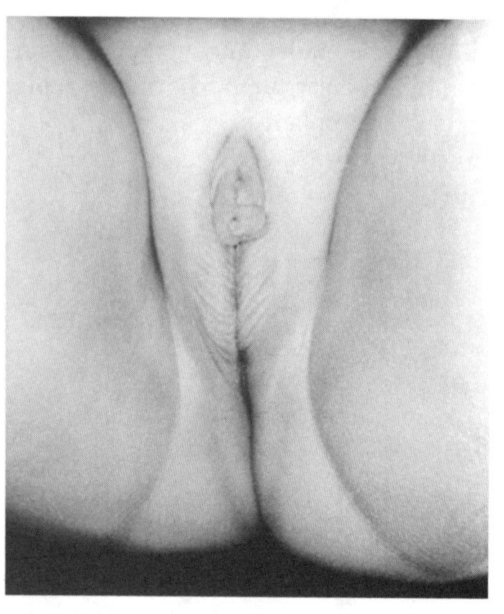

Figure 72-1. Physical exam findings.

Labs Karyotype: **46, XY. Müllerian structures absent;** inguinal swellings proved to be **maldescended dysgenetic testes.**

Imaging US: absence of müllerian structures and presence of dysgenic testes.

Micro Pathology Testes characterized by **seminiferous tubule degeneration** and invasion by connective tissue arranged in whorls.

NEPHROLOGY/UROLOGY

case 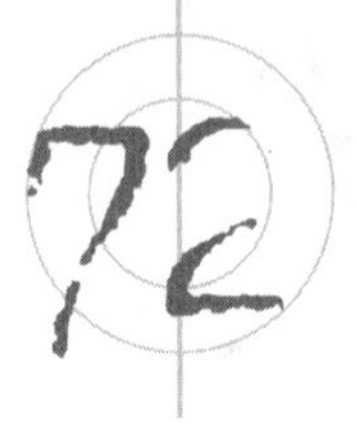

Testicular Dysgenesis

Differential

5α-Reductase deficiency
Androgen insensitivity syndrome
Congenital adrenal hyperplasia
3-β-Hydroxysteroid dehydrogenase deficiency

Discussion

The incidence of **gonadal tumors in dysgenetic gonads** may reach up to 30%, making orchiectomy and subsequent hormone replacement the best therapeutic option.

Treatment

Gonadectomy to protect against increased risk of testicular tumor; **hormone replacement** therapy given at puberty.

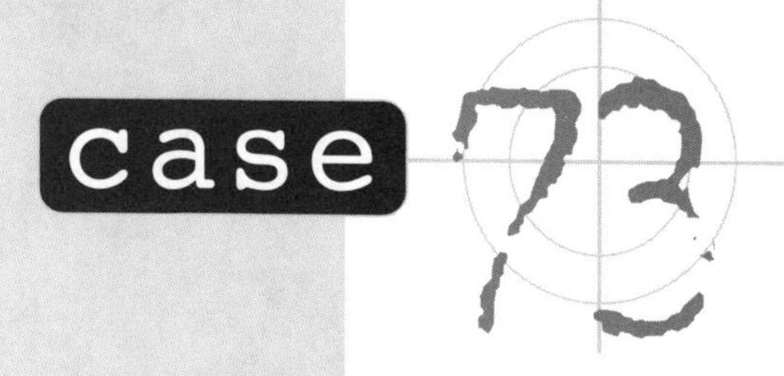

ID/CC A 23-year-old **white** man is seen by his family physician because of **dyspnea, bilateral enlargement of the breasts** (GYNECOMASTIA), and a **painless lump in the right testis** of approximately 2-month duration.

HPI He denies any history of STDs, genital ulcers, drug use, or trauma.

PE Bilateral nontender gynecomastia (due to increased hCG); left supraclavicular lymphadenopathy; 5-cm **hard mass** palpable **on right testis,** distorted shape; normal rectal exam.

Labs **Markedly elevated blood hCG and α-fetoprotein (AFP).**

Imaging US/MR, testes: **solid intratesticular mass** with some foci of hemorrhage (intratesticular masses usually malignant). CT, chest, abdomen, and pelvis (for staging disease): paracaval and interaortocaval lymphadenopathy.

Micro Pathology Cytotrophoblastic and syncytiotrophoblastic cells with hCG demonstrable within cytoplasm.

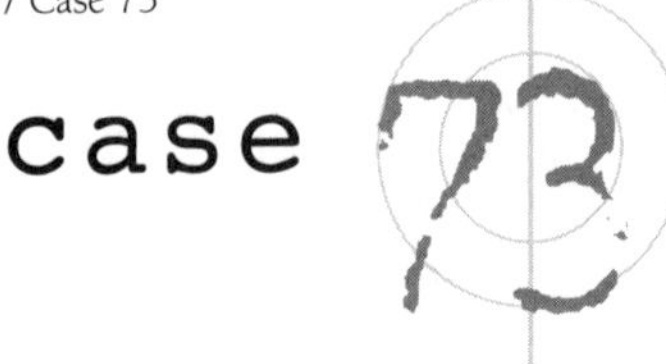

Testicular Teratoma (Mixed)

Differential

Epididymitis
Hydrocele
Testicular seminoma
Nonseminomatous testicular tumor
Testicular choriocarcinoma
Non-Hodgkin lymphoma

Discussion

Testicular cancer may be pure or mixed (mixed germ cell neoplasm) and is highly malignant with early and widespread metastasis. It is the most common neoplasm in men aged 20 to 35. Yolk sac tumors produce only AFP, whereas choriocarcinomas produce only hCG.

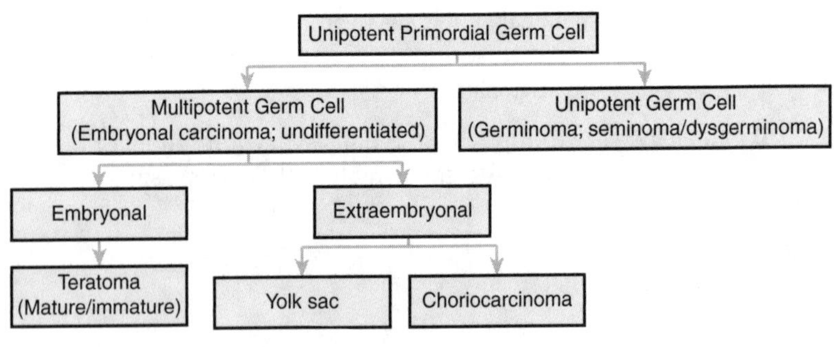

Figure 73-1. Differentiation of germ cell tumors.

Treatment

High radical inguinal orchiectomy followed by retroperitoneal lymph node dissection and cisplatin-based combination chemotherapy in selected cases.

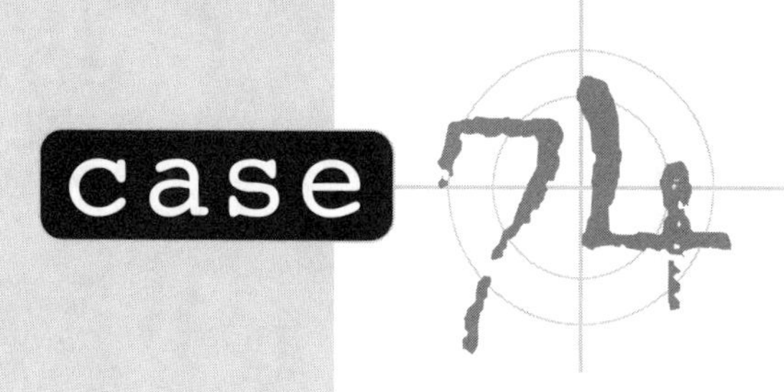

case 74

ID/CC A 9-year-old black boy is brought into the ER because of **sudden-onset** severe **pain** that he experienced in the lower abdomen and **scrotum** while playing soccer.

HPI He has no relevant medical history. Upon admission, he became nauseated and vomited three times.

PE Irritability; right **testicle tender, swollen,** and elevated; palpable normal epididymis anteriorly; **increased pain with elevation of mass** (PREHN SIGN); no hernia palpable; no transillumination of mass.

Labs UA: mild leukocytosis.

Imaging US, scrotum: asymmetric decreased color flow in testicle. Nuc-Tc99: **doughnut sign** (due to central testicular ischemia and circumferential collateral flow).

Gross Pathology Testicle markedly enlarged with hemorrhagic necrosis; scrotum may be purplish; cord twisted.

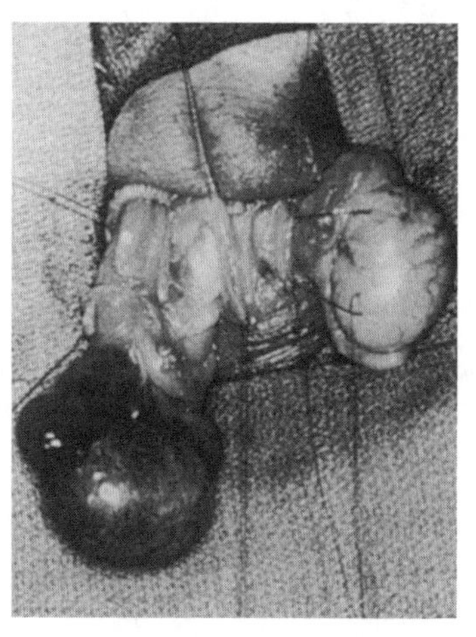

Figure 74-1. Gross pathology revealed during surgery.

Micro Pathology Severe venous congestion; interstitial hemorrhage; hemorrhagic necrosis.

NEPHROLOGY/UROLOGY

case 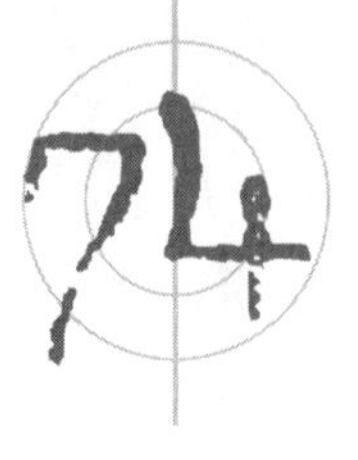

Testicular Torsion

Differential

Acute appendicitis
Epididymitis
Fournier gangrene
Orchitis

Discussion

Testicular torsion is a surgical emergency that needs to be differentiated from orchitis, epididymitis, and strangulated hernia. It is seen more frequently in an **undescended testicle** (CRYPTORCHIDISM); therefore, patients with cryptorchidism warrant close follow-up and perhaps corrective surgery.

Treatment

Immediate surgery (detorsion and fixation of testis to scrotum) due to risk of testicle loss (less than 4 hours); contralateral orchiopexy prophylactically (high incidence of bilaterality); atrophic testicle should be removed due to possible autoimmune destruction of contralateral testis.

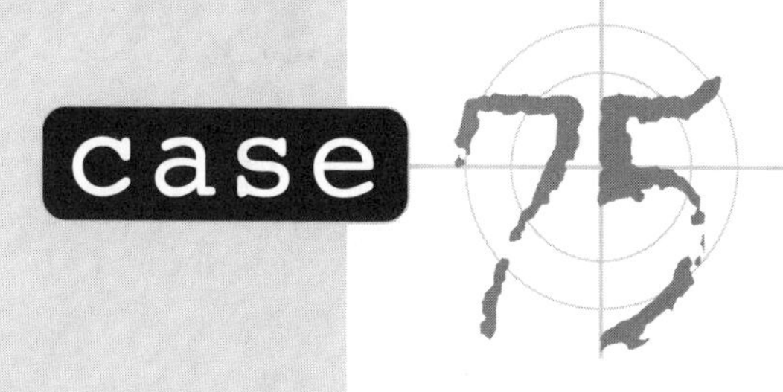

ID/CC A 45-year-old man with a high-grade **non-Hodgkin lymphoma** develops **oliguria, severe malaise, and fatigue** 36 hours following **chemotherapy treatment.**

PE Carpopedal **spasm** present; neither kidney is palpable; urinary bladder is empty.

Labs Lytes: hyperkalemia, **hyperuricemia**, and hyperphosphatemia with secondary hypocalcemia. **BUN and creatinine elevated.** UA: acidic urine with numerous **rhomboid crystals;** no casts or cells seen.

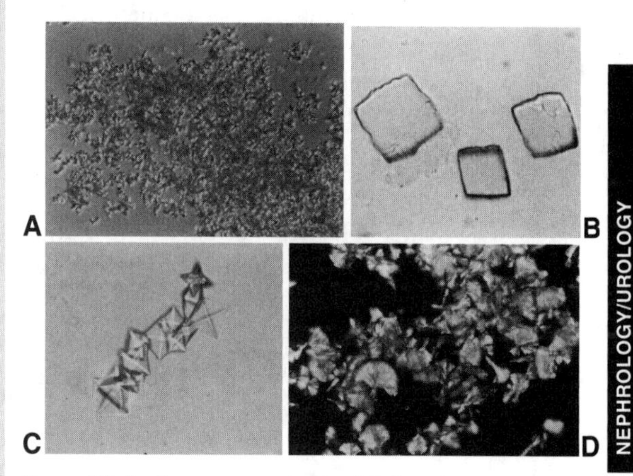

Figure 75-1. Numerous urate crystals in urine.

case 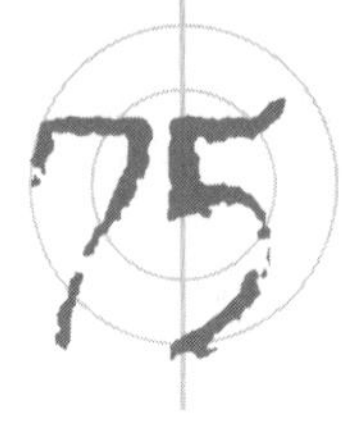

Urate Nephropathy

Differential

Fanconi syndrome
Urinary tract infection
Pyelonephritis
Calcium nephrolithiasis

Discussion

Tumor lysis syndrome is most often seen in patients with **lymphoma or leukemia** but is also seen in patients with a variety of solid tumors. The presence of a **large tumor burden, a high growth fraction, an increased pretreatment LDH level and uric acid level,** or pre-existing renal insufficiency increases the likelihood that a patient will develop tumor lysis syndrome. Increased levels of uric acid, xanthine, and phosphate may result in precipitation of these substances in the kidney. Renal sludging and acute renal insufficiency or failure further aggravate the metabolic abnormality.

Treatment

Maintenance of good hydration, brisk alkaline diuresis, and **pretreatment with allopurinol** are keys to prevention of this syndrome; once acute renal failure has developed, fluid and electrolyte balance must be maintained and dialysis may be necessary.

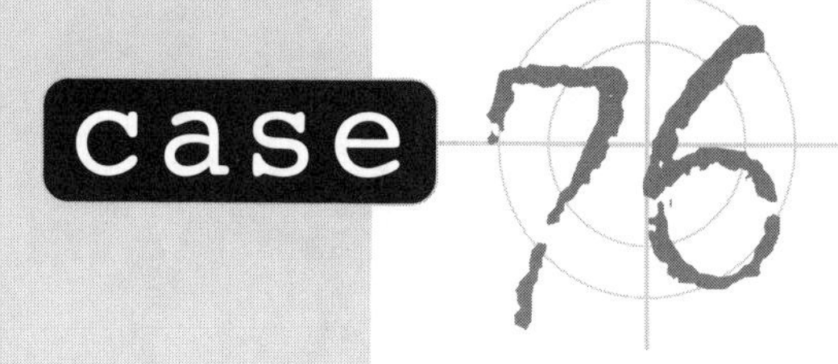

case 76

ID/CC A **3-year-old** boy is brought to his pediatrician for evaluation of an **abdominal mass** that his parents noticed.

HPI The child has been well all his life.

PE Slight pallor; weight and height within normal range; nontender, large, firm, and smooth intra-abdominal mass to right of midline; right **cryptorchidism** and **aniridia.**

Labs UA: microscopic **hematuria;** normal urinary vanillylmandelic acid (VMA); BUN increased; serum erythropoietin elevated.

Imaging IVP: displacement and distortion of right pelvicaliceal system. CT, abdomen: tumor arising from right kidney with areas of low density (due to necrosis); persistent ellipsoid area of enhancement (due to compressed renal parenchyma); no evidence of vascular invasion.

Gross Pathology Whitish, solid tumor with areas of hemorrhagic necrosis distorting normal renal parenchyma compressed into narrow rim.

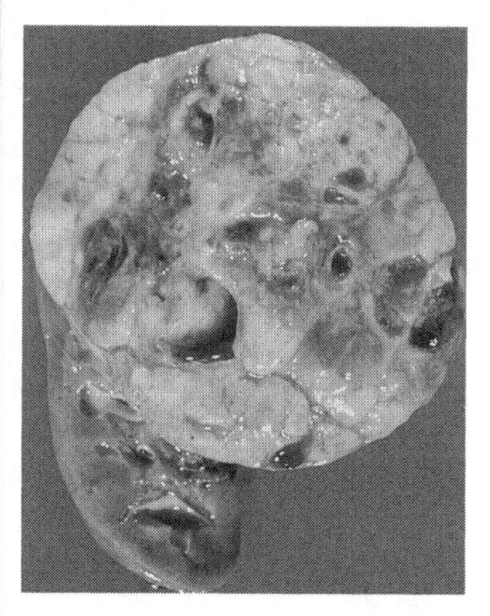

Figure 76-1. Large renal pole mass.

Micro Pathology Glomeruloid and tubular structures enclosed within spindle cell stroma; areas of cartilage, bone, or striated muscle tissue.

case 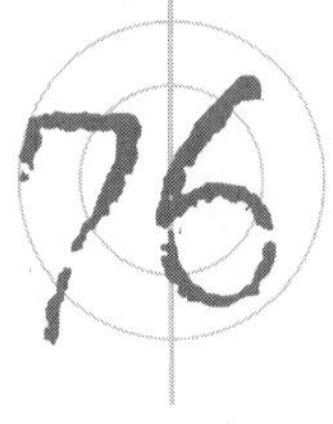

Wilms Tumor

Differential

Neuroblastoma
Juvenile polycystic kidney disease
Rhabdomyosarcoma
Dysplastic kidney

Discussion

Nephroblastoma (WILMS TUMOR) is a malignant tumor of embryonal origin. It is associated with deletions on **chromosome 11p** involving the WT-1 gene and should be differentiated from neuroblastoma and malignant lymphoma, which are other small cell tumors of childhood. Most cases are sporadic and are not associated with genetic syndromes or a positive family history. **WAGR syndrome** consists of Wilms tumor, aniridia, genitourinary abnormalities, and mental retardation.

Treatment

Surgical removal of kidney containing tumor; chemotherapy with actinomycin D and vincristine; radiotherapy.

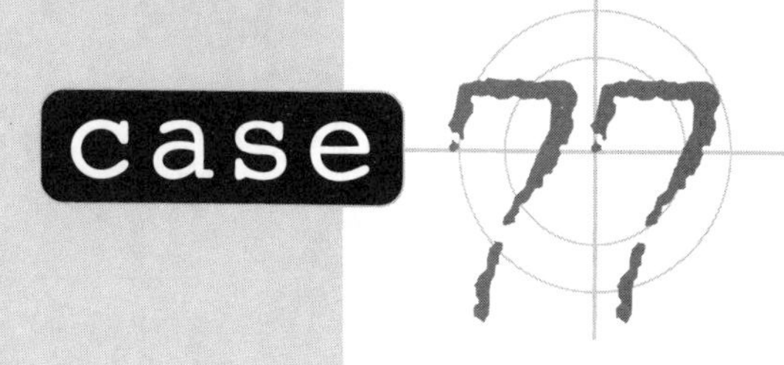

case 77

ID/CC A **14-year-old boy** is admitted to the hospital complaining of **pain** and **swelling** in the left **leg.**

HPI The pain has been present for 2 months but has become progressively worse over that period. There is no history of trauma or infection.

PE VS: **mild fever.** PE: tenderness and fusiform swelling over left femur.

Labs Elevated ESR. Karyotype: **translocation of the long arms of chromosomes 11 and 22.**

Imaging XR, left femur: lytic lesion in medullary zone of midshaft with cortical destruction and "**onion-skin**" appearance. CXR: no evidence of metastatic spread.

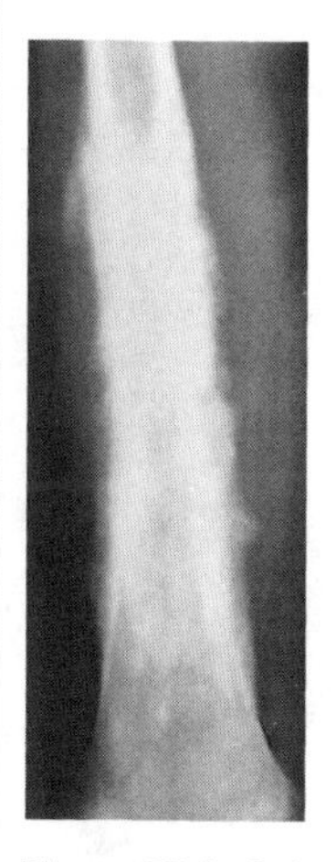

Figure 77-1. Onion skinning with cortical destruction.

Gross Pathology Large areas of bone lysis as tumors erode cancellous trabeculae of long bones outward to cortex.

Micro Pathology Biopsy of bone reveals sheets of uniform, small cells resembling lymphocytes; in many places tumor cells surround a central clear area, forming a "**pseudorosette.**" **Cell origin of tumor is unknown.**

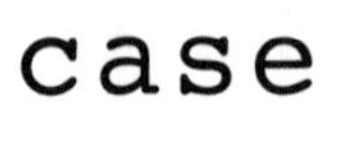

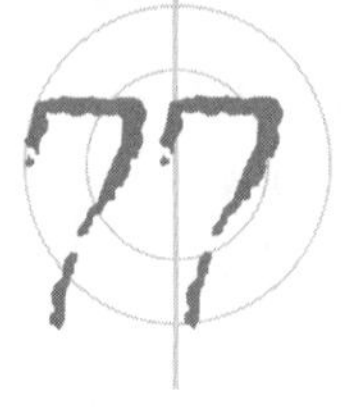

Ewing Sarcoma

Differential

Non-Hodgkin lymphoma
Osteomyelitis
Osteosarcoma
Rickets

Discussion

Diaphysis of the long bones is the **most common site of occurrence** of Ewing sarcoma. Five-year survival is 70% for locally resectable disease but only 30% for those with advanced metastasis.

Treatment

"Melt" tumor with radiotherapy; surgical resection; chemotherapy; regular follow-up for recurrence.

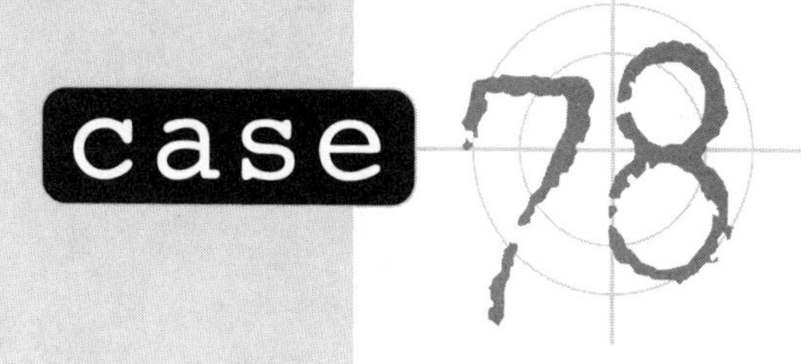

case 78

ID/CC A 45-year-old man visits an orthopaedist because of an **inability to extend his fifth fingers.**

HPI He has a long-standing history of **alcohol abuse** and has been to the ER several times for alcoholic gastritis.

PE Mild icterus; palmar erythema; muscle wasting; malnourishment; abdomen reveals 2+ ascitic fluid (due to alcoholic liver damage); **fifth fingers of left hand reveal flexion contracture** with nodular thickening and thick bands of tissue palpable upon drawing examining finger across palm.

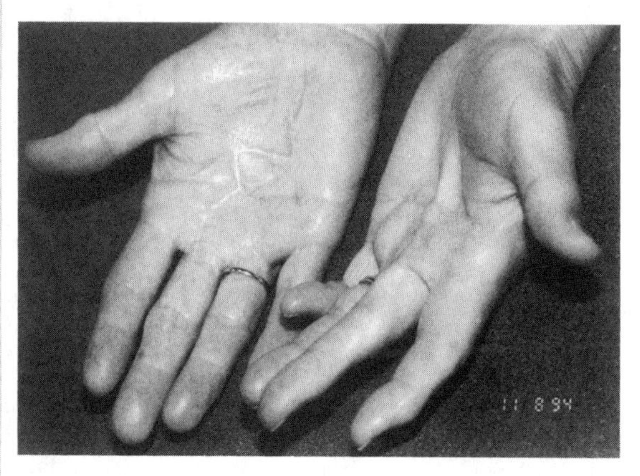

Figure 78-1. Extension deformity of the fifth digit.

Gross Pathology Infiltration of palmar fascia with fibrous tissue and subsequent contraction deformity.

Micro Pathology Infiltration of pretendinous fascia with myofibroblasts with fibrosis of pretendinous bands.

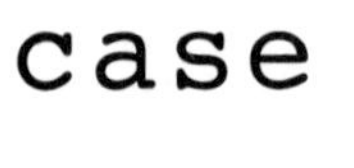
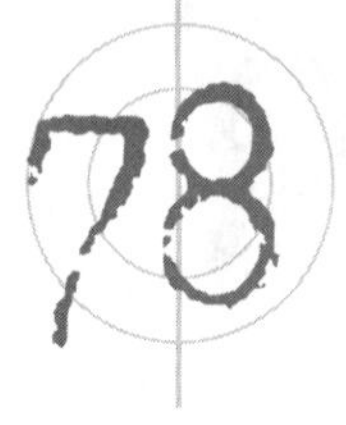

Dupuytren Contracture

Differential

Callus
Ganglion cyst
Tenosynovitis
Ulnar nerve palsy
Giant cell tumor of flexor tendon sheath

Discussion

Also called palmar fibromatosis, Dupuytren contracture is of unknown etiology but is associated with alcoholism and **manual labor.** It is associated with diabetes and anticonvulsant medications.

Treatment

Surgery (release of contractures and adhesions); frequently recurs.

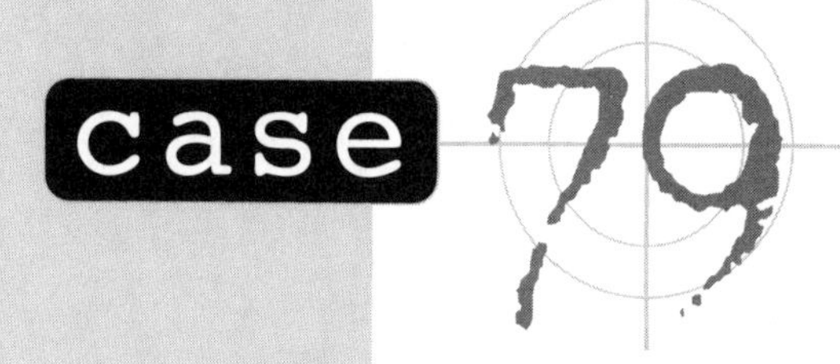

case 79

ID/CC A **60-year-old woman** is brought to the orthopaedic clinic with complaints of **pain in the left hip and inability to bear weight** on the left leg.

HPI **Three years** ago she sustained a **fracture of the neck of the femur** that was treated with external fixation. She is an **alcoholic** and has been taking **oral steroids** for many years for a chronic skin ailment.

PE All movements at left hip are restricted by pain; unable to bear weight on the limb.

Imaging XR, left hip: **increase in bone density of femoral head** and collapse of articular surface. MR, hip: more sensitive; decreased subchondral signal intensity and formation of reactive zones.

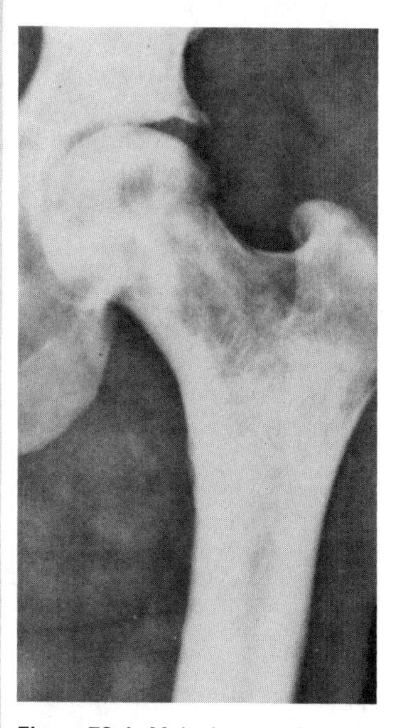

Figure 79-1. Molted areas of increased and decreased density of the femoral head.

case 79

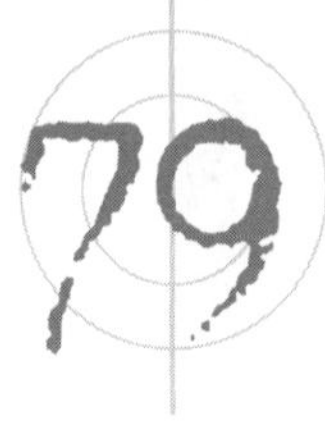

Avascular Necrosis of the Femoral Head

Differential

Bone metastasis
Osteomyelitis
Osteoporosis
Osteoarthritis

Discussion

Fracture of the neck of the femur is the most common cause of avascular necrosis of the femoral head; other risk factors include excessive alcohol consumption, steroid therapy, radiation therapy, sickle cell anemia, and deep sea diving **(Caisson disease).** Normally **blood is supplied to the head by three routes:** through vessels in the ligamentum teres, through capsular vessels reflected onto the femoral neck, and through branches of nutrient vessels within the substance of the bone. When the fracture occurs, nutrient vessels are necessarily severed, capsular vessels are injured to varying degrees, and **blood supply is maintained only through the vessels in the ligamentum teres.** This is a variable quantity and is often insufficient, resulting in avascular necrosis of the femoral head.

Treatment

Total hip replacement arthroplasty significantly reduces morbidity.

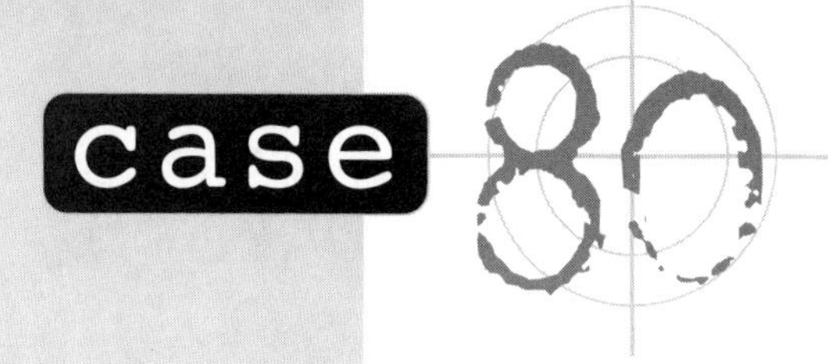

ID/CC A **12-year-old obese boy** is brought to the hospital with complaints of sudden-onset pain of the left hip along with a limp.

HPI The pain is felt in the left groin and often radiates to the left thigh and knee.

PE Left leg **externally rotated and about 2 cm shorter;** limited range of abduction and internal rotation; **upon flexing left hip, knee is drawn toward left axilla.**

Imaging XR, left hip (AP view): **growth plate widened and irregular.**

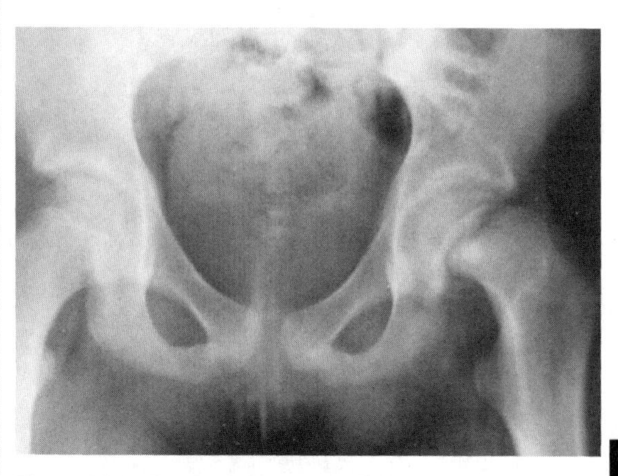

Figure 80-1. The femoral neck subluxates laterally and superiorly with respect to the epiphysis.

case 80

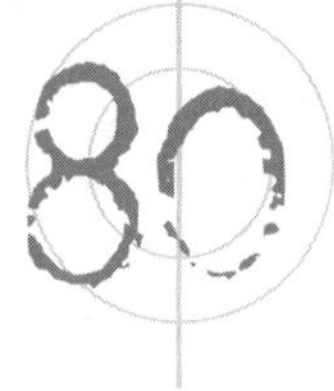

Slipped Capital Femoral Epiphysis

Differential

Juvenile rheumatoid arthritis
Legg–Calve–Perthes disease
Osgood–Schlatter disease
Septic arthritis
Sickle cell anemia

Discussion

Slipped femoral epiphyses affects youth **10 to 18 years old**, with boys more commonly affected than girls; affected children may be overweight and in some cases have delayed sexual development. Represents a Salter–Harris type I epiphyseal injury. Of cases, 25% are bilateral, of which 15% to 20% occur simultaneously. **Avascular necrosis** of the femoral head and **osteoarthritis** may arise as complications.

Treatment

Single-screw fixation.

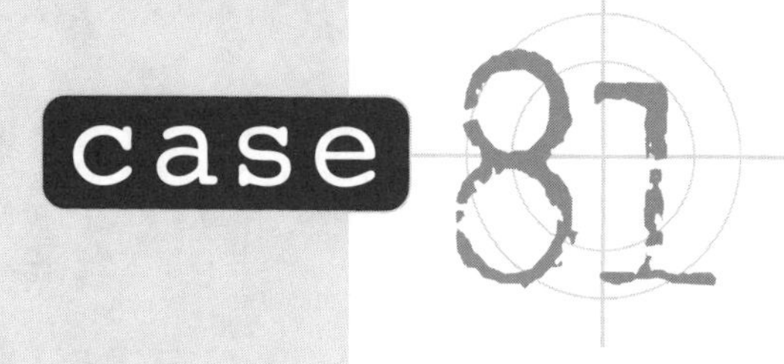

ID/CC A 25-year-old **athlete** is brought to the ER after she hurt her right knee.

HPI She had **fallen on a hyperextended right knee** that has been unstable since the fall. She recalls having heard a "popping" sound at the time of the injury.

PE Right knee exhibits effusion and **positive anterior "draw sign"** (tibia can be pulled forward on femur with knee flexed); instability of right knee joint (demonstrated by moving upper end of tibia forward on femur with knee flexed only 10 to 20 degrees; LACHMAN TEST).

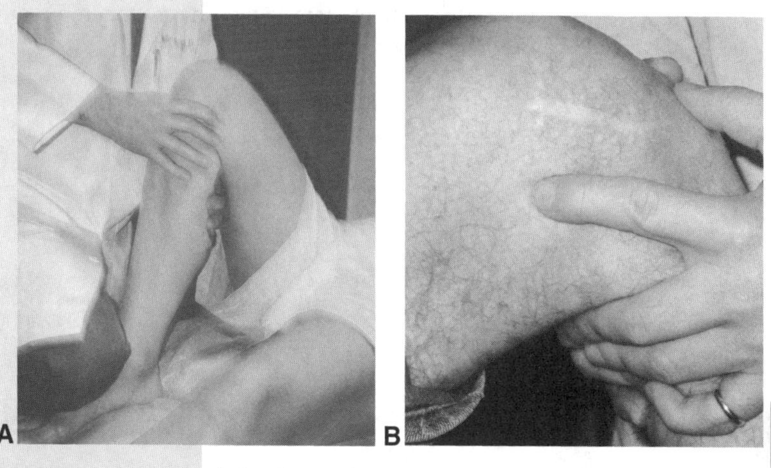

Figure 81-1. Positive anterior drawer sign.

Imaging MR, knee: indistinct, heterogeneous signal in expected region of the anterior cruciate ligament.

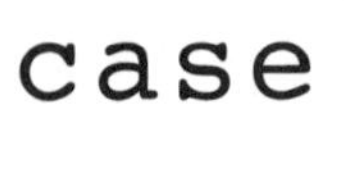
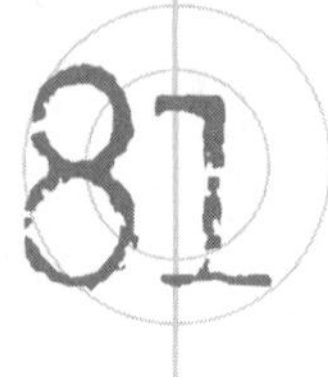

Anterior Cruciate Ligament Tear

Differential

Rheumatoid arthritis
Bursitis
Meniscal tear
Knee dislocation
Patellar tendon rupture

Discussion

The anterior cruciate ligament is torn by a force driving the upper end of the tibia forward relative to the femur or by hyperextension of the knee; the **posterior cruciate ligament is torn by a force driving the upper end of the tibia backward.**

Treatment

Surgical reconstruction for highly active patients; for less active patients, extensive physical therapy and avoidance of activity.

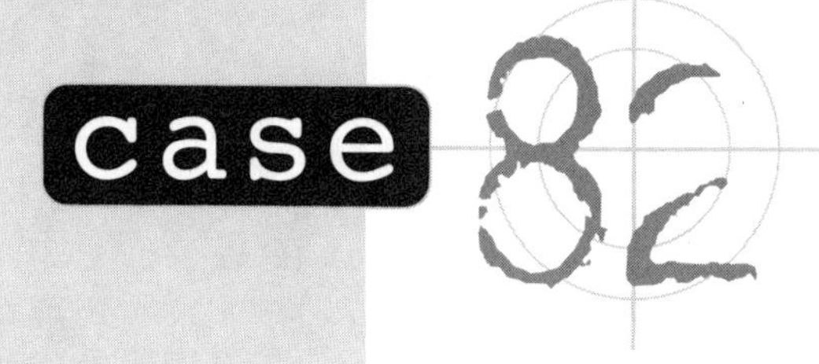

ID/CC A **60-year-old obese woman** is seen with complaints of gradually progressing **stiffness and pain after use of the right knee.**

HPI The pain and stiffness are accompanied by swelling and deformity of the joint. She also reports difficulty walking and limitation of movement.

PE Tenderness, pain, and crepitus of right knee on motion; firm swelling (caused by underlying bony proliferations) and joint effusion; fixed deformities: bony enlargement and a varus angulation, causing limited motion at joint; hands show **bony swellings on distal interphalangeal joints** (HEBERDEN NODES).

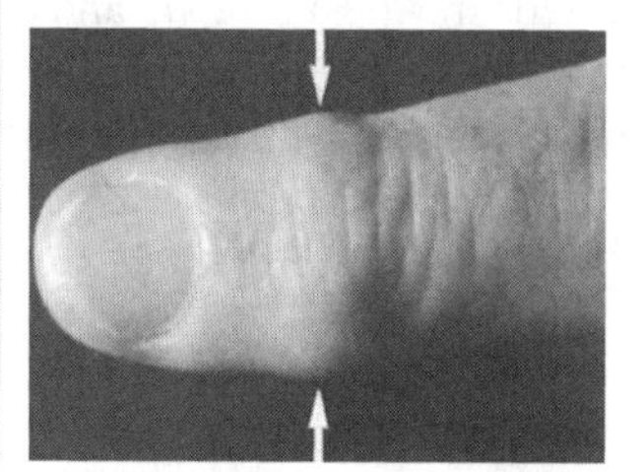

Figure 82-1. Hard dorsolateral nodules on the DIP joints.

Labs Synovial fluid shows no evidence of inflammation; normal viscosity and mucin clot tests; protein, glucose, and complement levels also normal; serum rheumatoid factor not raised.

Imaging XR, right knee (AP and lateral views): narrowing of joint space (medial > lateral); subchondral bone sclerosis; subchondral cysts and osteophytes.

Gross Pathology Late stages of the disease show **eburnation** of joint surface, **remodeling** of joint surface, **osteophytes** around lateral margins of joint, subchondral bone cysts, and bone sclerosis.

Micro Pathology Loss of articular cartilage, bone resorption, and irregular and variable new bone and cartilage formation.

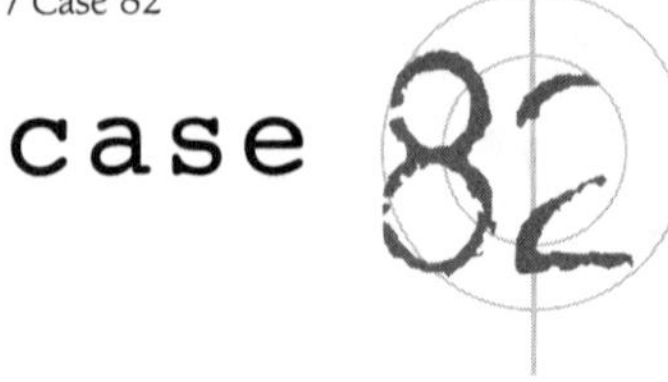

Osteoarthritis

Differential

Ankylosing spondylitis
Gout
Pseudogout
Psoriatic arthritis
Reactive arthritis

Discussion

Osteoarthritis, a degenerative joint disease, is characterized by the degeneration of articular cartilage and by progressive destruction and remodeling of the joint structures. The condition affects large weight-bearing joints such as the knees, hips, and lumbar and cervical vertebrae; other joints commonly affected are the PIP, DIP, and first carpometacarpal joints. It is more common in women, and its incidence increases with age, particularly after 55.

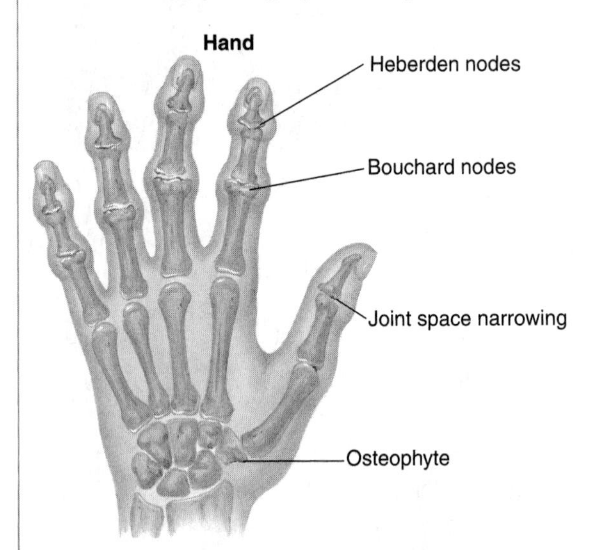

Figure 82-2. Hand joint findings in osteoarthritis.

Treatment

Pain relief, improvement of mobility, and correction of deformity; joint replacement.

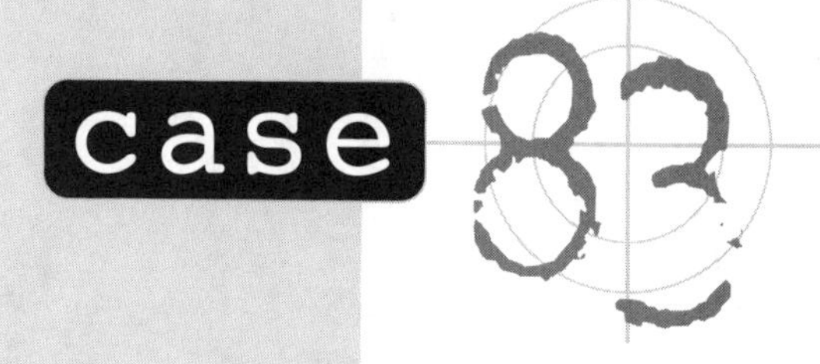

case 83

ID/CC A **12-year-old boy** presents with a **swelling** above the right knee and associated pain.

HPI There is **no history of trauma** at the site of pain. There has been **no discharge** from the swollen region and **no fever.**

PE **Bony-hard,** tender, roughly circular swelling above right knee **(distal femur)**; mechanical restriction of movement of right knee.

Labs Normal ESR; **elevated serum alkaline phosphatase** (may be used as marker of treatment response).

Imaging XR, plain: osteoblastic bone lesion at distal end of femur; periosteal elevation by metaphyseal tumor (CODMAN TRIANGLE).

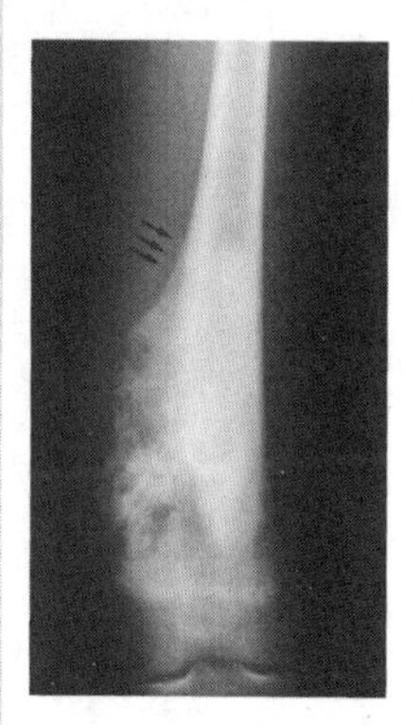

Figure 83-1. Ill-defined destructive lesion with an extensive soft tissue component. Codman triangles are present (arrows).

Gross Pathology Firm, whitish mass with **osteoblastic** bone sclerosis originating from **metaphysis** adjacent to epiphyseal growth plate and invading through cortex, lifting up periosteum.

Micro Pathology Bone biopsy shows multinucleated giant cells, anaplastic cells with pleomorphism, and osteoid production with foci of sarcomatous degeneration.

case 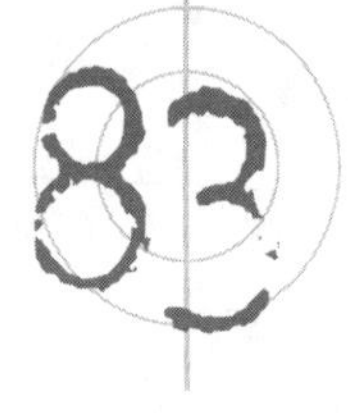

Osteosarcoma

Differential

Ewing sarcoma
Histiocytosis
Osteomyelitis
Stress fracture
Bone cyst

Discussion

Osteogenic sarcoma is the most common primary malignant tumor of bone (excluding myeloma and lymphoma); it may be osteoblastic or osteolytic. Pathologic fractures may occur; pulmonary metastases are frequent. There is an increased risk with Paget disease, prior radiation, and hereditary retinoblastoma.

Treatment

Surgical amputation with total joint prosthesis or complex bone reconstruction; consider limb salvage; radiotherapy, chemotherapy.

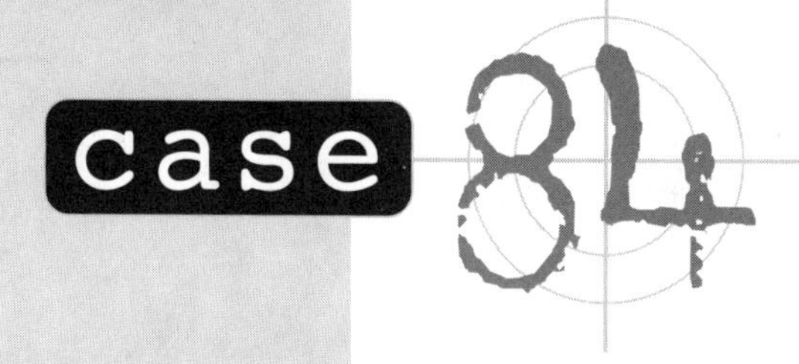

case 84

ID/CC A 70-year-old immigrant from England presents with **pain** in his right leg, producing an awkward gait, along with bilateral **hearing loss.**

HPI He has also noted a progressive **increase in his hat size.**

PE Slight **bowing of right tibia;** normal rectal exam; mixed conductive and **sensorineural hearing loss** confirmed by audiometry; physical exam otherwise normal.

Labs **Markedly elevated alkaline phosphatase;** mildly elevated serum calcium and phosphorus; normal serum transaminases; **increased urinary excretion of hydroxyproline.**

Imaging XR, skull: scattered **islands of bone lysis** (OSTEOPOROSIS CIRCUMSCRIPTA); mixed **thickening** (blastic) **and lucency** (lytic lesions) of bone (COTTON WOOL APPEARANCE).

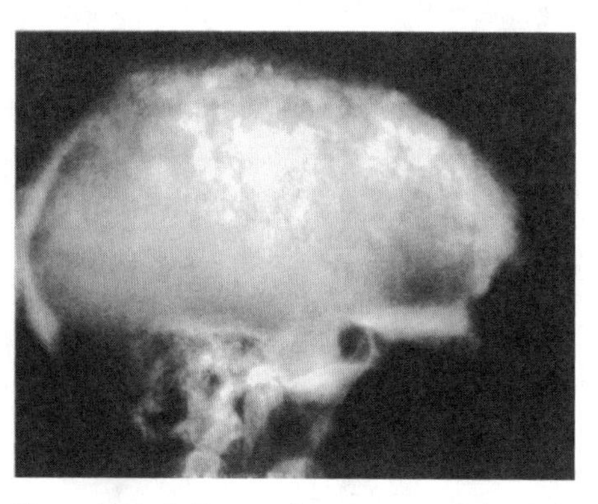

Figure 84-1. Cotton wool appearance of the skull.

Gross Pathology Expansion of bone cortex, blastic bone lesions, and bowing of long bones (thick ivory bones).

Micro Pathology Multiple cement lines with unmineralized osteoid; indicative of excessive osteoblastic and osteoclastic activity.

case 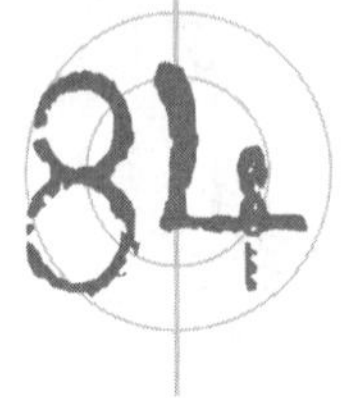

Paget Disease of Bone

Differential

Osteoarthritis
Osteoporosis
Osteomalacia
Acromegaly
Bone metastasis

Discussion

A condition of probable viral etiology, Paget disease is characterized by osteoclastic destruction of bone initially with excessive osteoblastic repair, producing bone sclerosis. When extensive, the resulting increased blood flow leads to **high cardiac output congestive heart failure.** Other complications are **pathologic fracture and osteosarcoma** (1% of patients).

Treatment

Medical treatment with bisphosphonates (inhibit osteoclastic activity), calcitonin; surgical treatment with total joint arthroplasty, nerve decompression, and osteotomies.

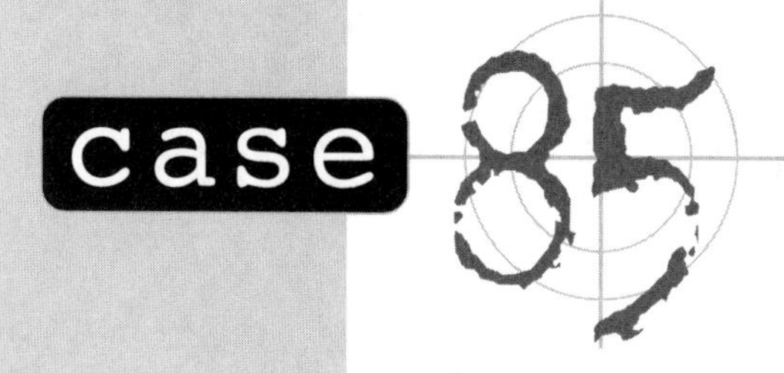

ID/CC A **5-year-old boy** is brought to a physician with sudden-onset progressive severe **pain, swelling, and redness** of the right knee joint.

HPI He has had a **high-grade fever** for the past 2 days. A few days ago he **injured his right leg, and the injury subsequently became infected**; he is now unable to move his right leg properly.

PE VS: fever. PE: infected wound on right leg; right **knee red, swollen, and tender;** all movements restricted by pain.

Labs CBC: **neutrophilic leukocytosis** with shift to the left. Elevated ESR; **synovial fluid (obtained following joint aspiration) opaque and yellowish; joint effusion has WBC count >50,000/L;** Gram stain reveals **Gram-positive cocci in clusters**.

Imaging XR, right knee: early, soft tissue swelling and joint effusion; late, articular erosions and reactive sclerosis. NUC, gallium scan: increased uptake by right knee joint.

case

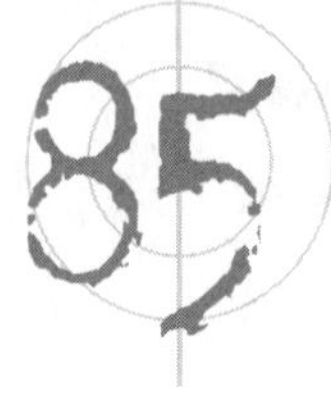

Septic Arthritis—Staphylococcal

Differential

Juvenile rheumatoid arthritis
Reactive arthritis
Kawasaki disease
Lyme disease
Septic bursitis

Discussion

Septic arthritis is caused by pyogenic organisms and is more common among children, especially males. *Staphylococcus aureus* is the most common cause; other organisms include streptococci, gonococci, pneumococci, and *Neisseria meningitidis*. Organisms reach the joint via hematogenous routes (most common; the primary focus may be a pyoderma, throat infection, IV drug use, etc.), secondary to adjacent osteomyelitis, or via penetrating wounds, or the condition may be iatrogenic.

Treatment

Broad-spectrum parenteral antibiotics initially, then specific antibiotics following culture sensitivity reports; if necessary, joint may be opened, washed, and closed with a suction drain and immobilized until signs of inflammation subside.

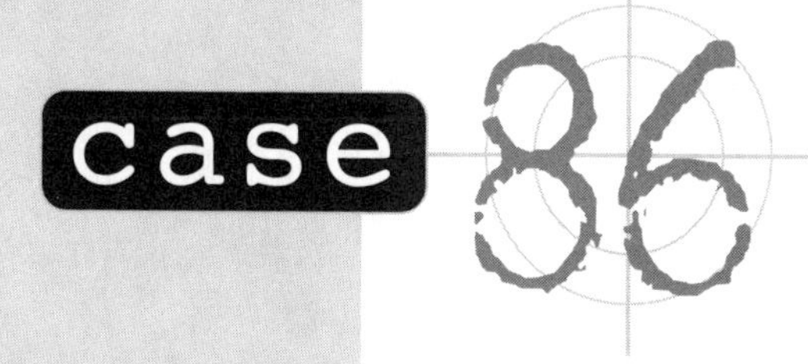

case 86

ID/CC A 55-year-old woman presents with an **aching pain in the back of her neck,** a feeling of stiffness, and a **"grating" sensation upon movement.**

HPI She also has a history of a vague, ill-defined, and ill-localized pain spreading over her shoulder region.

PE Neck **slightly kyphotic; posterior cervical muscles tender; neck movements** slightly **restricted at extremes** due to pain; **audible crepitation on movement; diminished supinator and biceps reflex in the left upper limb;** no motor or sensory loss demonstrable.

Imaging XR, cervical spine (lateral view): **narrowing of intervertebral disk space with formation of osteophytes at vertebral margins,** especially anteriorly.

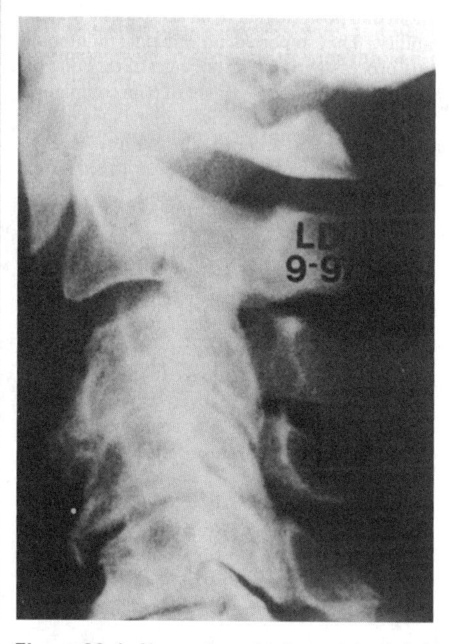

Figure 86-1. Narrowing of intervertebral disk space with formation of osteophytes at vertebral margins.

case 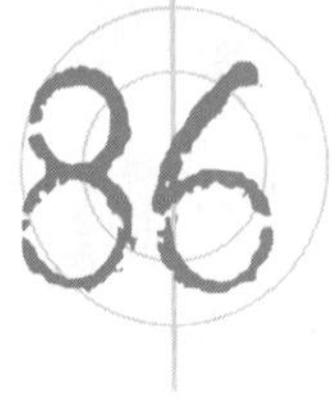

Cervical Spondylosis

Differential

Central cord syndrome
Cervical myofascial pain
Brachial plexopathy
Cervical disk disease
Brown–Sequard syndrome

Discussion

Degenerative arthritis occurs predominantly in the **lowest three cervical joints**. The changes **first affect the central intervertebral joints and later affect the posterior intervertebral (facet) joints. Osteophytes commonly encroach on the intervertebral foramina,** reducing the space for transmission of the cervical nerves. If the restricted space is further reduced by the traumatic edema of the contained soft tissues, manifestations of nerve pressure are likely to occur. Rarely, the spinal cord itself may suffer damage, producing a cervical myelopathy.

Treatment

There is a strong tendency for the **symptoms of cervical spondylosis to subside spontaneously.** Treatment includes **analgesics, physiotherapy, and support of the neck** by a closely fitting collar of plaster or plastic. Surgical intervention is required for patients who are unresponsive to conservative therapy as well as for those with progressive myelopathy or radiculopathy.

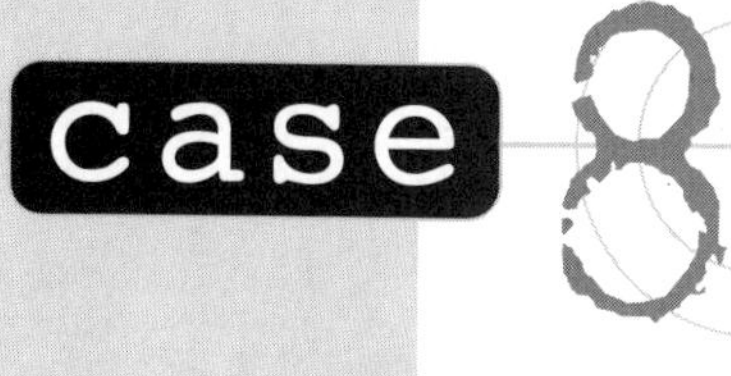

ID/CC An asymptomatic **60-year-old** white **man** undergoing a routine physical exam is discovered to have a **pulsating abdominal mass.**

HPI The patient has a history of **occasional abdominal pain** and **hypercholesterolemia** that has been poorly controlled by diet and medication.

PE **Pulsating, painless upper abdominal mass** approximately 5 cm in diameter.

Imaging KUB, lateral: calcification of aneurysm wall. CT/US, abdomen: dilated aorta with irregular calcified wall; large, eccentric mural thrombus seen.

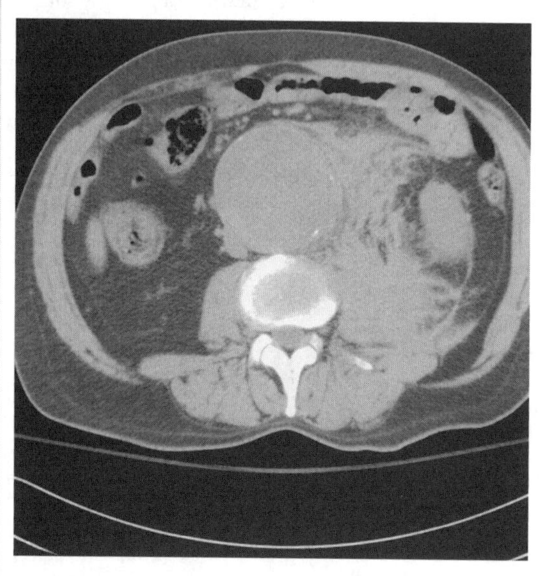

Figure 87-1. An 8.3-cm infrarenal dilation of the aorta.

Gross Pathology Most aneurysms are located between renal arteries and iliac bifurcation; thrombus may also be present; intramural dissection may also be seen.

Micro Pathology Aneurysm wall contains all three layers (intima, media, adventitia) ("TRUE" ANEURYSM).

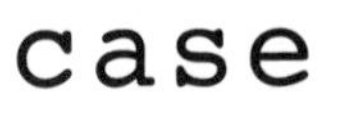
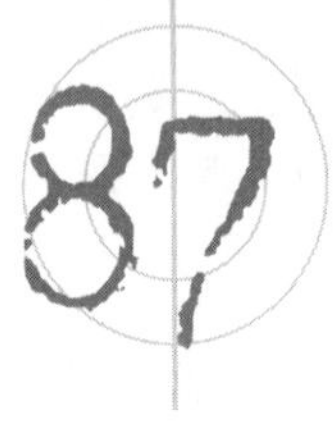

Abdominal Aortic Aneurysm

Differential

Acute appendicitis
Diverticular disease
Pancreatitis
Myocardial infarction
Small bowel obstruction

Discussion

The risk of rupture with potentially fatal bleeding increases with size. Abdominal aortic aneurysm is usually caused by **atherosclerotic** disease and is often associated with coronary artery disease. It may also be caused by trauma, infection (e.g., syphilis), **cystic medial degeneration**, and arteritis. Sequelae include rupture, embolization, infection, vascular occlusion secondary to thrombus formation, and compression of adjacent structures (e.g., ureters, vertebrae).

Treatment

Surgical replacement with graft (if >5.5 cm or symptomatic); consider endovascular stent/graft.

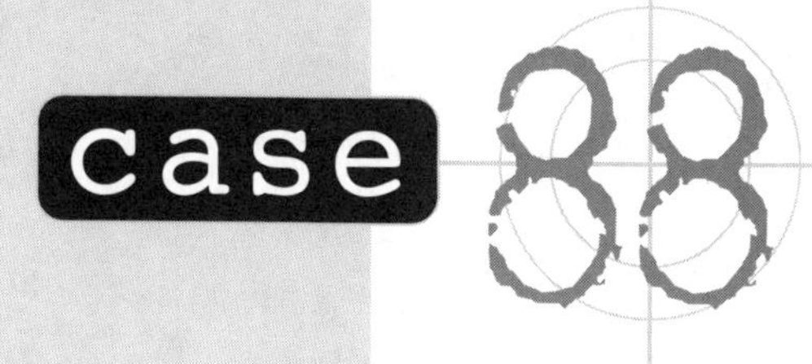

ID/CC A **42-year-old** white **woman**, the **mother of five**, develops **acute intermittent pain in the right upper quadrant** and right scapula **after eating a fatty meal.**

HPI She is of **Native American ancestry** and is 30 pounds **overweight.** She also complains of **nausea** and has **vomited** three times. She has had several prior episodes of similar pain following meals.

PE VS: fever; tachycardia. PE: **obese;** tenderness in right upper abdominal quadrant with **inspiratory arrest on palpation** (MURPHY SIGN); hypoactive bowel sounds.

Labs Hypercholesterolemia. CBC: **leukocytosis with mild neutrophilia.** Elevated direct bilirubin; **elevated alkaline phosphatase.**

Imaging US: distended gallbladder with **wall thickening** containing **multiple echogenic shadows** (stones). Nuc, HIDA: failure to visualize gallbladder indicates cystic duct obstruction by stone.

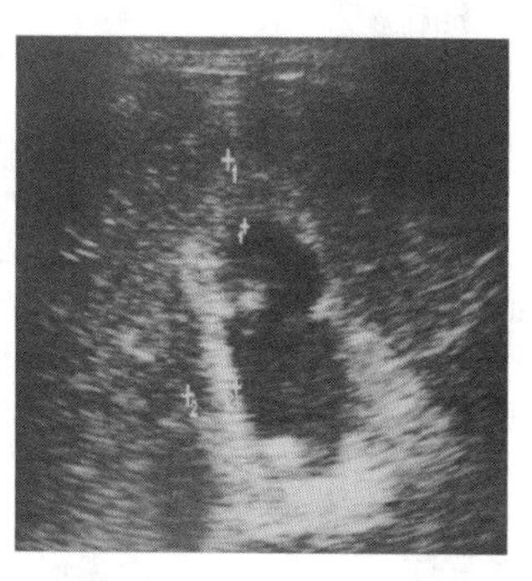

Figure 88-1. Ultrasonography demonstrating echogenic foci and gallbladder wall thickening.

Gross Pathology Gallbladder inflammation with wall edema to acute gangrene with necrosis, pus formation, and perforation with peritonitis.

Micro Pathology Gallbladder mucosa contains lipid-laden foamy macrophages.

case

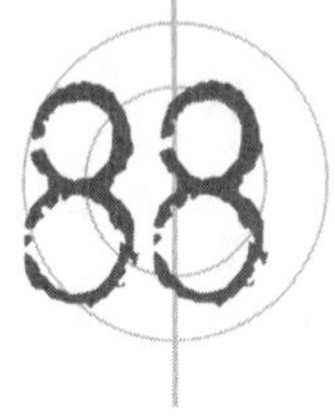

Acute Cholecystitis

Differential

Appendicitis
Pancreatitis
Perforated peptic ulcer
Pyelonephritis
Myocardial infarction
Right lower lobe pneumonia

Discussion

Although calculi are involved in most cases of acute cholecystitis, **acalculous** cases arise after nonbiliary major surgeries, severe trauma or burns, and sepsis and in the postpartum state. Most stones are composed of **cholesterol;** less common are **pigmented stones** made principally of unconjugated bilirubin and calcium salts.

Breakout Point

Clinical risk factors of cholecystitis include the **four F's**
Fat
Female
Forty
Fertile

Treatment

Initial conservative treatment with IV fluids, analgesics, and antibiotics followed by elective **cholecystectomy** (usually laparoscopic) is definitive.

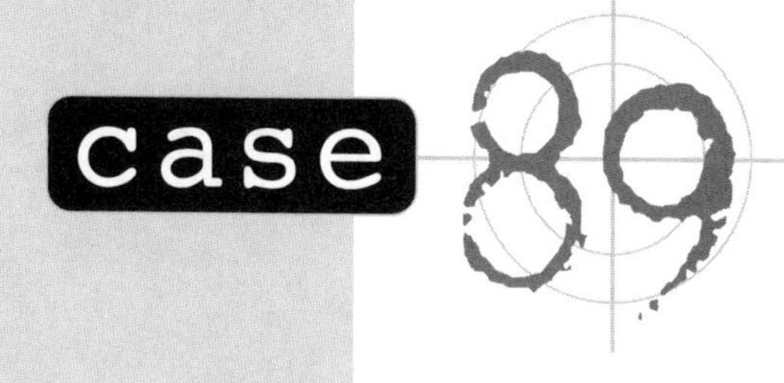

ID/CC A 17-year-old student presents with **anorexia** and poorly localized **periumbilical pain followed by nausea** and two episodes of **vomiting.**

HPI Four hours after presentation, the **pain shifted to the right lower quadrant** and he developed a **low-grade fever.**

PE VS: mild tachycardia; low-grade fever. PE: **right lower quadrant tenderness with guarding and rebound;** pain in right lower quadrant when pressure applied to left lower quadrant (ROVSING SIGN); **pain localized to junction of outer and middle third of the line from anterior superior iliac spine to umbilicus** (MCBURNEY POINT); right lower quadrant pain elicited by passive hip flexion (PSOAS SIGN) and by passive internal and external rotation of hip (OBTURATOR SIGN).

Labs CBC: **elevated WBC count; predominance of neutrophils.** Normal serum amylase. UA: normal.

Imaging KUB: right psoas shadow blurred; generalized ileus with air-fluid levels; increased soft tissue density in right lower quadrant; small radiopaque **fecalith** in right lower quadrant. US: **noncompressible tubular structure** in right lower quadrant. CT, abdomen: enlarged appendix with enhancement of appendiceal wall and periappendiceal fat stranding.

Gross Pathology Early lesion: hyperemic appendix with fibrinous exudate; late lesion: purulent exudate with necrosis and perforation; fecalith occasionally present.

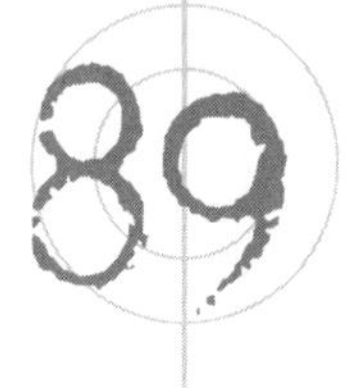

Appendicitis

Differential

Cholecystitis
Diverticular disease
Mesentary ischemia
Pelvic inflammatory disease (female)
Ovarian torsion
Gastroenteritis

Discussion

The peak incidence of appendicitis is in the second and third decades. Causes include **obstruction by fecaliths** (33%) and **lymphoid hyperplasia** (60%); it is occasionally caused by tumors (carcinoid tumor is the most common tumor of the appendix), parasites, foreign bodies, and Crohn disease. Complications include perforation, **periappendiceal abscess,** peritonitis, and generalized or wound sepsis.

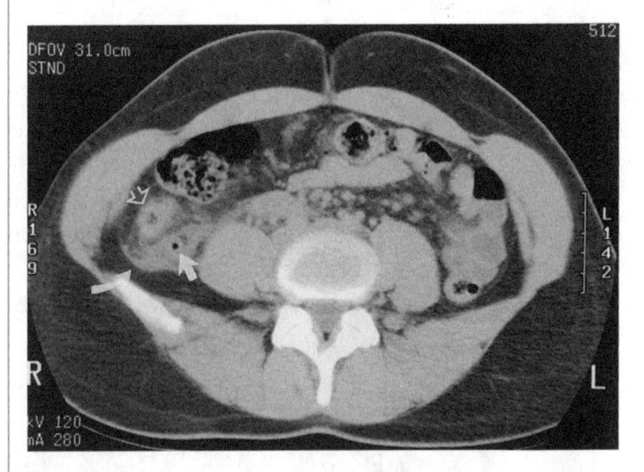

Figure 89-1. Enlarged, thickened appendix (open arrow), surrounding fat stranding and inflammation (curved arrow) and extraluminal air, implying perforation (closed arrow).

Treatment

Appendectomy with preoperative antibiotic coverage.

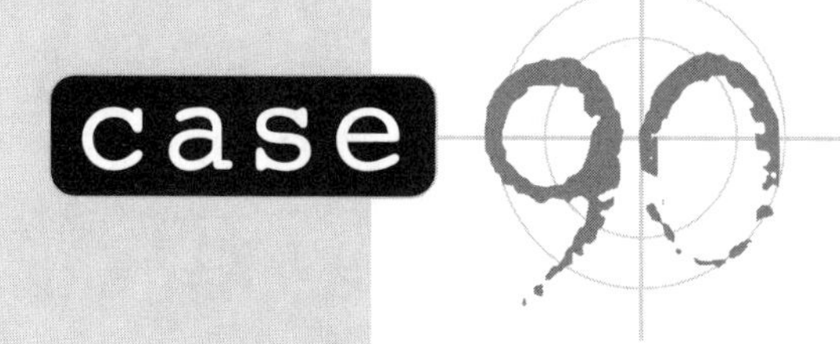

ID/CC A **67-year-old** white woman complains of increasing fatigue for several months.

HPI She has also noticed significant **weight loss** and **intermittent diarrhea.**

PE Marked **pallor;** palpable left supraclavicular lymph node (VIRCHOW NODE); palpable mass in right iliac fossa; hepatomegaly.

Labs CBC/PBS: microcytic, hypochromic **anemia. Positive stool guaiac test;** elevated serum carcinoembryonic antigen (CEA) levels.

Imaging BE: large, irregular fungating mass in cecum. US: metastatic hepatic nodules. Colonoscopy: large fungating growth in cecum.

Gross Pathology **Cauliflower-like, fungating, nonobstructing growth** in cecum; may be polypoid, sessile, or constricting.

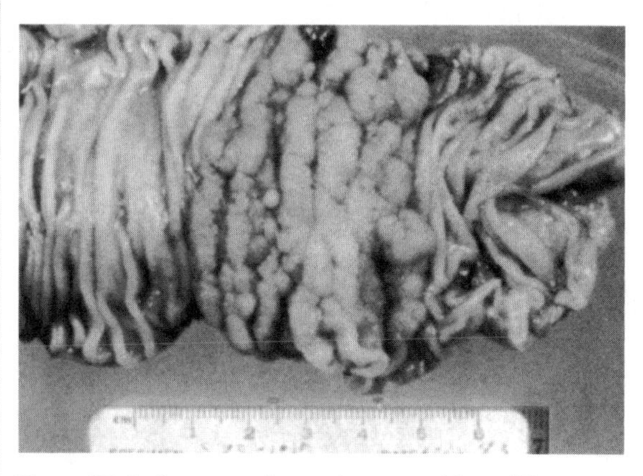

Figure 90-1. Gross specimen of cecum with cauliflower-like fungating mass.

Micro Pathology Well-differentiated adenocarcinoma.

case 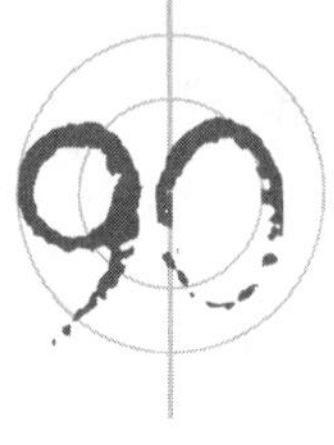

Cecal Carcinoma

Differential

Diverticular disease
Cecal volvulus
Intussusception
Myocardial infarction
Colonic angiodysplasia

Discussion

Starting at age 50, colon cancer screening with colonoscopy and fecal occult blood testing is recommended for the average-risk population.

Treatment

Right hemicolectomy with regional lymph node dissection for staging; adjuvant chemotherapy in selected patients; follow-up for recurrence by monitoring CEA levels.

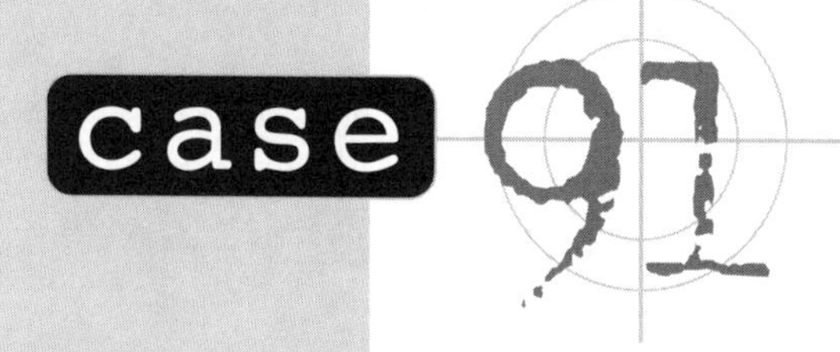

ID/CC A 68-year-old **black man** presents with anorexia, progressive **dysphagia**, odynophagia, and **weight loss.**

HPI The patient has been drinking very **hot tea** since he was 11 years old and **smokes** one pack of cigarettes per day. His history also reveals heavy **alcohol** intake; occasional cough, vomiting, and **regurgitation;** and severe dysphagia with **solids, progressing to liquids.**

PE Emaciation; fixed, **nonpainful supraclavicular node;** pale conjunctiva.

Labs CBC/PBS: hypochromic, microcytic anemia. Hemoccult-positive stool; hypoalbuminemia.

Imaging EGD: **irregular fungating esophageal mass** in middle third of esophagus with partial obstruction. CT, chest: irregular esophageal mass with invasion of mediastinum and enlarged para-aortic lymph node.

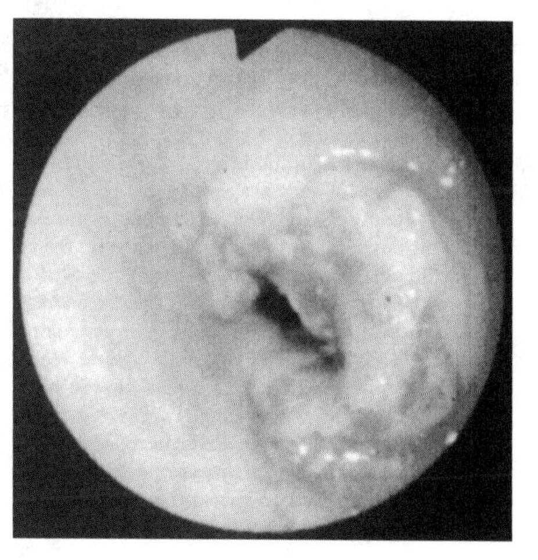

Figure 91-1. Exophytic luminal mass.

Gross Pathology Large fungating mass protruding toward esophageal lumen.

Micro Pathology Squamous cell carcinoma on biopsy.

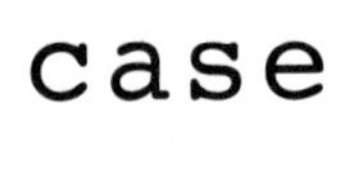
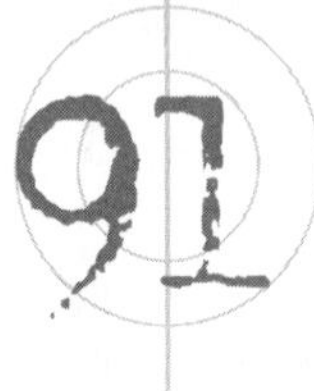

Esophageal Carcinoma

Differential

Achalasia
Esophageal stricture
Hiatal hernia
Schatzki ring
Esophagitis

Discussion

The most common variant of esophageal carcinoma is **squamous cell carcinoma (SCC),** which is associated with alcohol and tobacco use and is more common in blacks. Although the incidence of SCC is decreasing in the United States, the incidence of adenocarcinoma is rising dramatically and is more common in whites with **Barrett** syndrome (glandular metaplasia of the squamous epithelium of the distal esophagus is caused by chronic, untreated gastroesophageal reflux disease).

Treatment

Laser ablation of tumor with palliative stent placement; palliative radiotherapy; surgical resection followed by chemotherapy plus radiotherapy for curable tumors; eventual gastrostomy tube placement.

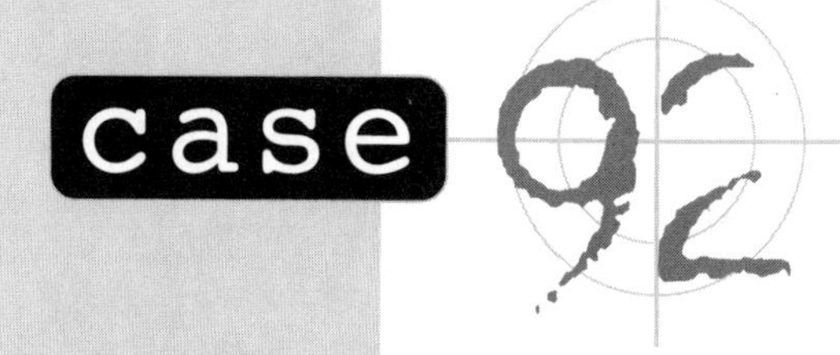

ID/CC	An 83-year-old white man complains of **anorexia, frequent vomiting**, and a **gnawing midepigastric pain** of several-month duration.
HPI	The pain is **not relieved by antacids or milk.** The patient has **lost significant weight** over the past few months due to diarrhea after every meal.
PE	Pale, **emaciated** male in moderate distress; left supraclavicular lymph node (VIRCHOW NODE) palpable.
Labs	CBC: **hypochromic, microcytic anemia.** Stool **positive for occult blood**; LFTs normal.
Imaging	UGI: large fungating lesion on greater curvature of stomach with fistulous tract running to transverse colon. EGD: same.
Gross Pathology	Polypoid, raised, fungating mass projecting into lumen; situated at distal end of stomach.
Micro Pathology	Biopsy reveals a **well-differentiated adenocarcinoma** with **signet-ring** cells.

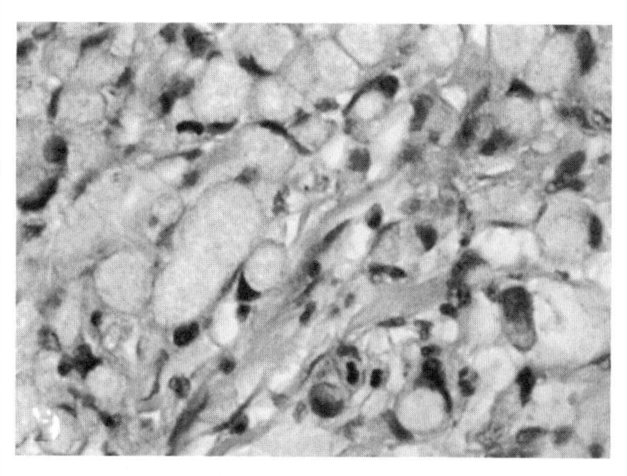

Figure 92-1. Signet ring cells.

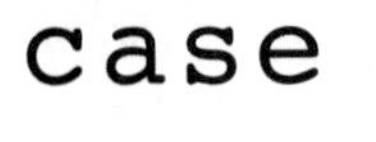

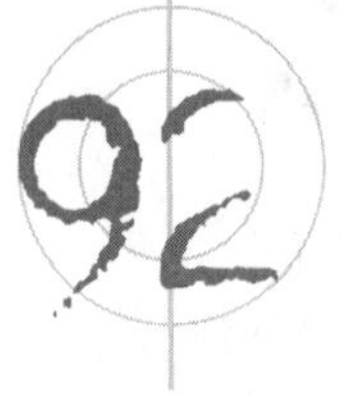

Gastric Carcinoma

Differential

Esophageal cancer
Gastric ulcer
Chronic gastritis
Non-Hodgkin lymphoma
Gastroenteritis

Discussion

Most commonly found on the **lesser curvature** in the **antrum** and **pyloric areas**, adenocarcinomas may be one of two types: **intestinal** and **diffuse.** Chronic atrophic gastritis, pernicious anemia, infection with *Helicobacter pylori*, postsurgical gastric remnants, and type A blood are all predisposing risk factors for the development of adenocarcinoma. It most commonly spreads hematogenously to the liver and may spread transperitoneally to the ovaries (KRUKENBERG TUMOR).

Treatment

Esophagogastrectomy for tumors of the cardia and gastroesophageal junction; subtotal gastrectomy for tumors of the distal stomach; radiotherapy; chemotherapy.

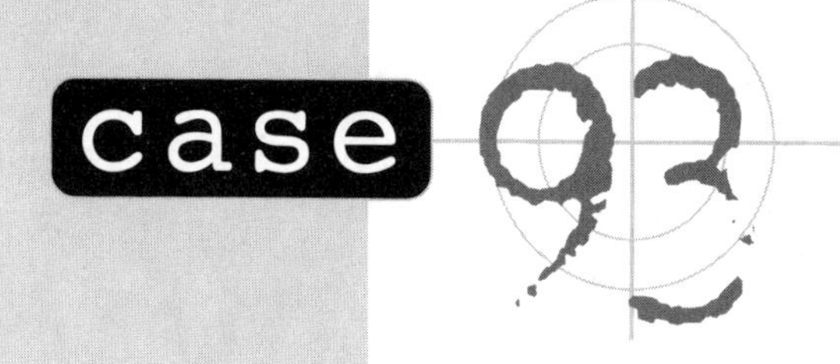

ID/CC A 44-year-old man is admitted to the hospital following episodes of **vomiting blood** (HEMATEMESIS) and passing **black, tarry, foul-smelling stools** (MELENA).

HPI He has experienced **recurrent painless hematemesis** and **melena** for several years, but repeated evaluations have been negative.

PE Pallor.

Labs CBC: **microcytic, hypochromic anemia.** Nasogastric aspirate has **coffee-ground** appearance.

Imaging UGI/EGD: 5-cm mass in fundus of stomach with 2-cm ulcer on surface.

Gross Pathology Postoperative specimen reveals a firm, circumscribed nodular **mass within the gastric wall** covered by mucosa.

Micro Pathology Whorling interlaced bundles of spindle-shaped cells; no evidence of anaplasia.

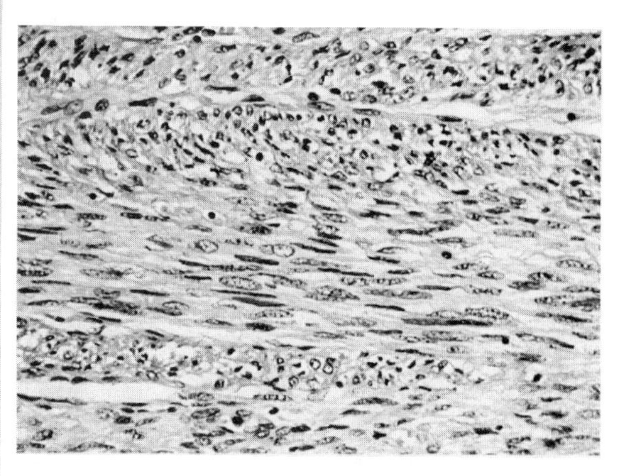

Figure 93-1. Smooth muscle cells intertwined in bundles.

case 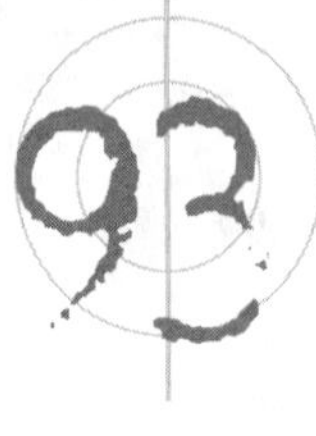

Gastric Leiomyoma

Differential

Gastric carcinoid
Angiosarcoma
Gastric lymphoma
Lipoma
Metastatic melanoma

Discussion

Gastric leiomyoma is the **most common benign tumor of the stomach.**

Treatment

Surgical resection.

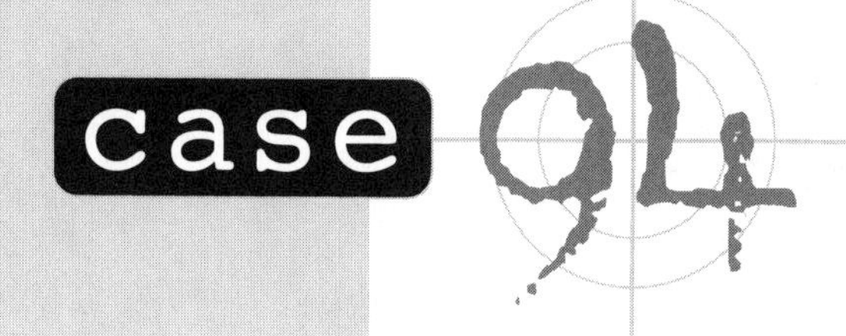

ID/CC A 40-year-old man presents with **cramping abdominal pain** and **vomiting** of 3-hour duration.

HPI He also complains of an **inability to pass stool or flatus** (OBSTIPATION) for the past 3 days. Two years ago, he underwent an emergency appendectomy for a ruptured appendix.

PE Dehydration; **abdominal distention;** generalized mild tenderness over abdomen without rebound or guarding; bowel sounds heard as **high-pitched tinkles during pain paroxysms;** empty rectal vault on rectal exam.

Labs CBC/PBS: leukocytosis with hemoconcentration. Serum amylase levels normal.

Imaging XR, abdomen: "stepladder" pattern of multiple **dilated loops of small bowel** and **multiple air–fluid levels; colon and rectum gasless** (air in colon or rectum would indicate an intestinal ileus); no free air under diaphragm.

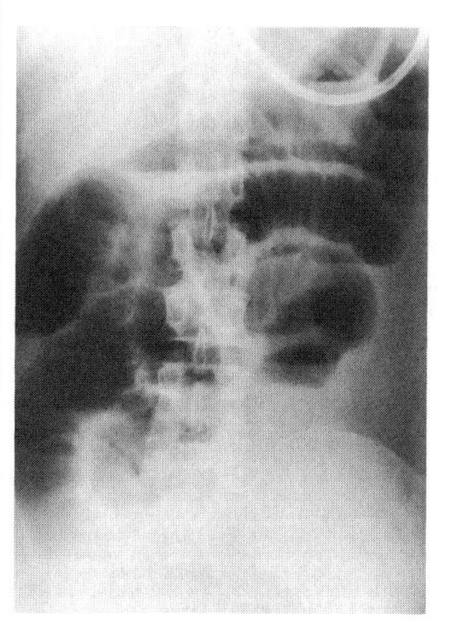

Figure 94-1. Upright film shows multiple air–fluid levels in dilated small bowel.

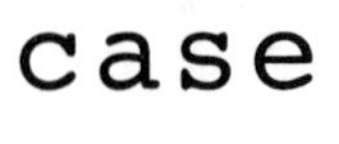

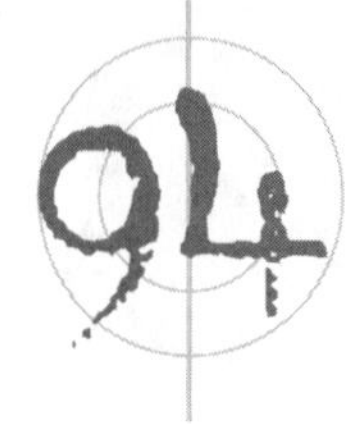

Intestinal Obstruction—Acute

Differential

Appendicitis
Constipation
Mesenteric ischemia
Diverticular disease

Discussion

The most common causes of small bowel obstruction are intestinal **adhesions secondary to prior abdominal surgery, intussusception**, **volvulus**, and incarcerated **hernia**; the most common causes of large bowel obstruction are **carcinoma**, **volvulus**, and **sigmoid diverticulitis.** Complications include **strangulation** and **necrosis** of the bowel wall leading to perforation, peritonitis, sepsis, and shock.

Treatment

IV fluid and electrolyte replacement; nasogastric suction/decompression; broad-spectrum antibiotics; surgery.

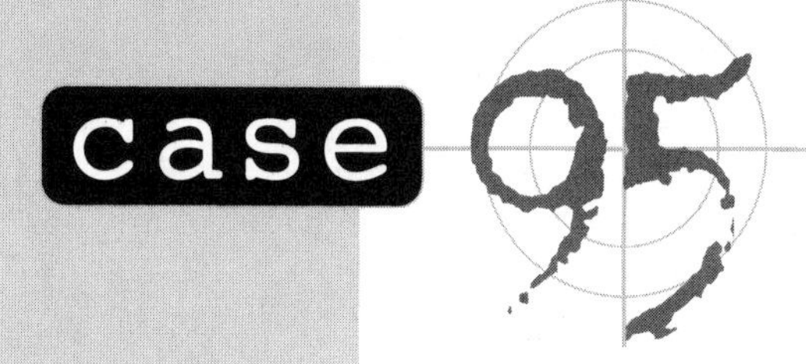

ID/CC An **18-month-old boy** is brought to the ER by his parents because of acute, **intermittent abdominal pain,** abdominal distention, and passage of "**red currant jelly" stools.**

HPI The child had previously been well, and his immunization schedule is complete. He **vomited** twice following admission.

PE Child crying and screaming, with knees drawn to abdomen; abdomen tender and distended; **oblong** (sausage-shaped) **mass** in abdomen (most often in right upper quadrant) that hardens with palpation; examining finger stained with **mucus and blood** on digital rectal examination.

Labs No parasites on stool exam; no pathogen on stool culture.

Imaging XR, abdomen: gas in small intestine and absence of cecal gas shadow. BE: **telescoping** of ileum into cecum.

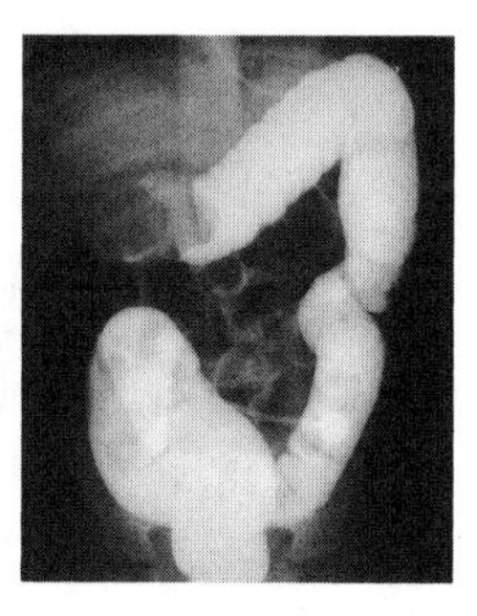

Figure 95-1. Telescoping of one bowel segment into another as event by barium enema.

Gross Pathology During operation, three layers are seen: entering or inner tube, returning or middle tube, and sheath or outer tube.

Micro Pathology **Ischemic necrosis** with sloughing of mucosa, producing "red currant jelly" stools.

case

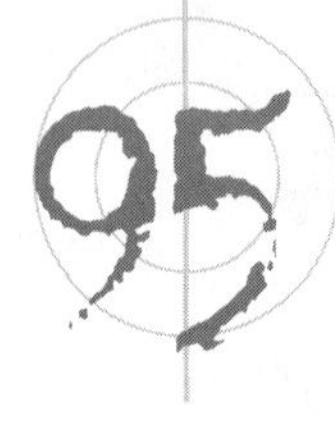

Intussusception

Differential

Appendicitis
Volvulus
Incarcerate hernia
Gastroenteritis

Discussion

Of cases of intussusception, 95% are idiopathic and usually originate near the ileocecal junction. The condition is associated with adenovirus infections, which produce **hyperplasia of Peyer patches** in the terminal ileum, which serves as a nidus for intussusception. It is also seen with **lead points** (e.g., Meckel diverticulum, polyps, parasites, duplications, hemangiomas, and suture lines).

Treatment

Hydrostatic (barium) or pneumatic (air) **reduction** using an enema; surgical reduction or resection if that fails or is contraindicated owing to perforation or gangrene.

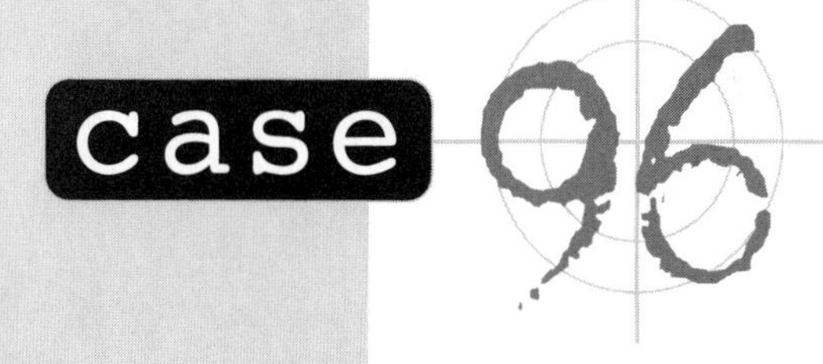

ID/CC A 51-year-old man complains of **pruritus** and **abdominal pain** that **radiates to his back** along with **significant weight loss.**

HPI He also states that his **urine is dark** and that his **stools are clay-colored** (ACHOLIC). He admits to a history of **smoking** (60 pack-years) and heavy alcohol use with **multiple prior bouts of pancreatitis.**

PE **Cachectic** male; **scleral icterus** (indicates **jaundice**); **hepatomegaly; palpable gallbladder** (COURVOISIER SIGN).

Labs **Markedly elevated direct bilirubin** (20 mg/dL); absence of urinary urobilinogen; markedly **elevated alkaline phosphatase; elevated carcinoembryonic antigen (CEA) and CA 19-9.**

Imaging CT/US: **mass in head of pancreas; dilated intrahepatic bile ducts.** ERCP: abrupt cutoff of main pancreatic duct. UGI: narrowed lumen of duodenum.

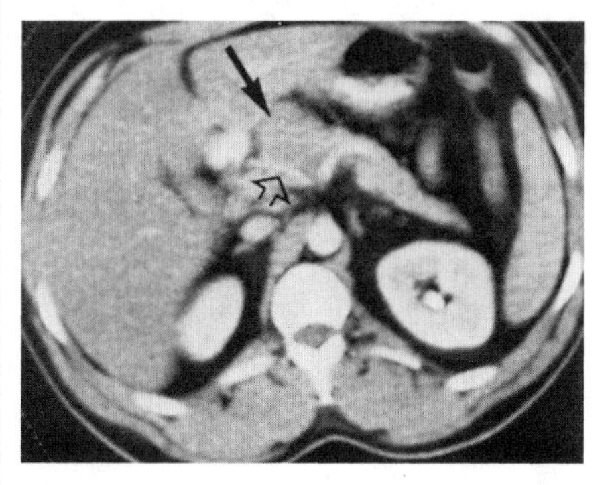

Figure 96-1. Mass in the head of the pancreas (dark arrow).

Gross Pathology Hard nodular mass with ill-defined borders invading pancreatic parenchyma and **obstructing common bile** duct around head of pancreas.

Micro Pathology Pancreatic mass biopsy reveals a poorly differentiated **ductal adenocarcinoma** in clusters.

case 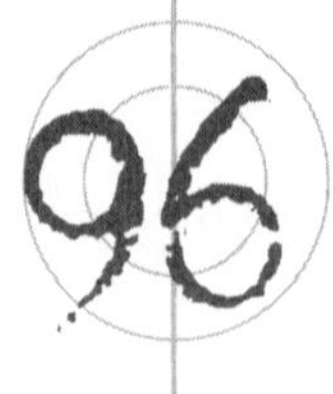

Pancreatic Carcinoma

Differential

Abdominal aortic aneurysm
Ampulla carcinoma
Chronic pancreatitis
Neoplasm of the endocrine pancreas

Discussion

Chronic gallbladder disease, diabetes mellitus, hereditary pancreatitis, **chronic pancreatitis, cigarette smoking,** diets high in meat and fat, and occupational exposure to **carcinogens** are predisposing factors. Pancreatic carcinoma carries a **poor prognosis** (85% are already locally invasive or metastatic at the time of diagnosis) and is associated with a mutation in the K-ras oncogene and the p53 tumor suppressor gene. Complications include hypercoagulability (resulting in **migratory thrombophlebitis**, also known as the Trousseau sign).

Treatment

Surgical pancreaticoduodenectomy (WHIPPLE PROCEDURE); chemotherapy; supportive and palliative care (biliary decompression to relieve jaundice; celiac plexus block for pain).

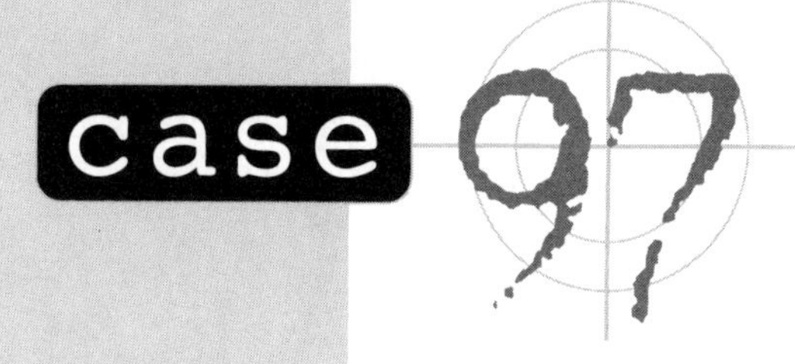

case 97

ID/CC A term newborn girl is noted to have **edema, dyspnea, cyanosis, and marked jaundice.**

HPI Her **mother is blood type** AB **Rh-negative**. Her **previous childbirth** was an uneventful full-term vaginal delivery conducted outside the United States 4 years ago. The mother **did not receive any subsequent immunizations.**

PE Pallor; **marked jaundice**; hypotonia; **S3 and S4**; hepatosplenomegaly; **generalized edema.**

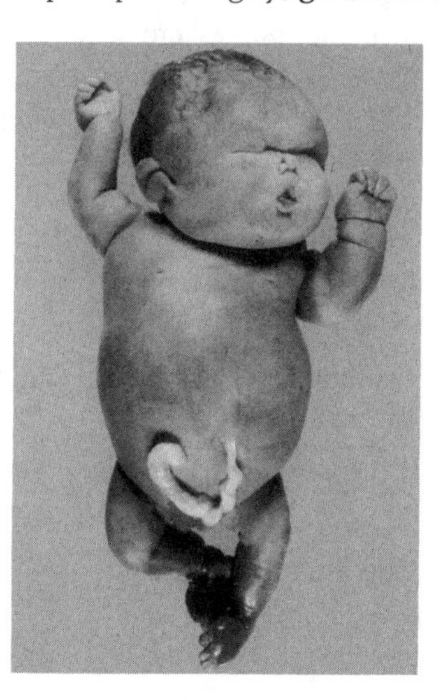

Figure 97-1. Severe hydrops.

Labs Blood type of **mother** AB **Rh-negative;** blood type of father A Rh-positive; **blood type of first child** A **Rh-positive**. Mother's serum: **positive** indirect **Coombs test,** anti-D antibody titer >1:64. Neonate's serum: positive direct Coombs test, increased indirect bilirubin.

Gross Pathology Brain specimen from autopsy reveals yellow staining of basal ganglia by unconjugated bilirubin (KERNICTERUS).

case 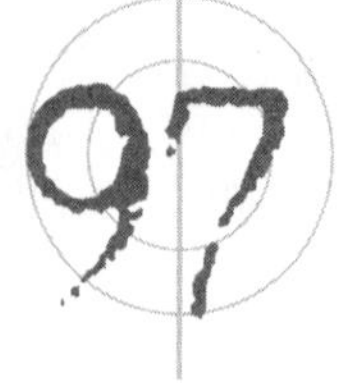

Erythroblastosis Fetalis

Differential

Cytomegalovirus infection
Parvovirus B19 infection
Hypothyroidism
Congenital syphilis
Toxoplasmosis

Discussion

The mother produced anti-D (IgG) antibodies owing to her exposure to D antigen during her delivery of an Rh-positive infant. In her subsequent pregnancy, these antibodies crossed the placenta and reacted with the fetus's RBCs (Rh-positive), producing hemolysis and **fetal heart failure with generalized edema** (HYDROPS FETALIS). To prevent Rh isoimmunization, all Rh-negative mothers with an Rh-positive fetus should receive **RhO (D) immune globulin** following deliveries, abortions, ectopic pregnancies, or even amniocentesis.

Treatment

Phototherapy (promotes elimination of bilirubin); exchange transfusion.

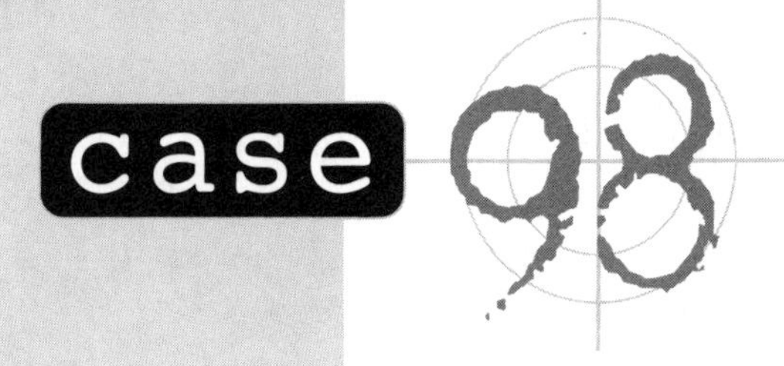

ID/CC	Paramedics are called at 7:00 A.M. because a **2-month-old boy,** the child of African immigrants, cannot be awakened by his mother; upon arrival, it is clear that the child has been dead for at least 4 hours.
HPI	The child was slightly premature, but aside from this, his history was unremarkable. There was nothing that could directly explain the episode. On directed history, **the mother admits to being a smoker and remembers that the child had a URI 4 days ago.**
PE	No pathologic cause revealed that could explain death.
Gross Pathology	Autopsy reveals petechiae on pleural and pericardial surfaces, pulmonary congestion, and scattered foci of lymphocytic tissue in interstitium of lungs.

case 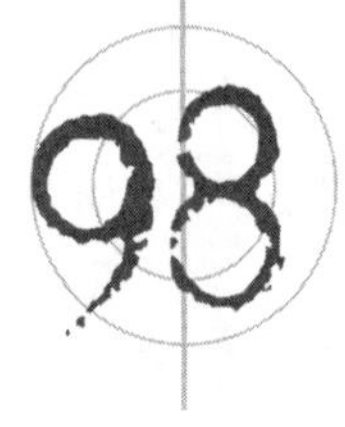

Sudden Infant Death Syndrome

Differential

Congenital cardiac anomalies
Bronchiolitis
Hypoplastic left heart
Child abuse/neglect
Long-chain acyl-CoA dehydrogenase deficiency
Sleep apnea

Discussion

Sudden infant death syndrome (SIDS) refers to **death of an infant under 1 year** of age, usually during sleep, in which **death remains unexplained** even after complete autopsy; most have a history of minor URIs.

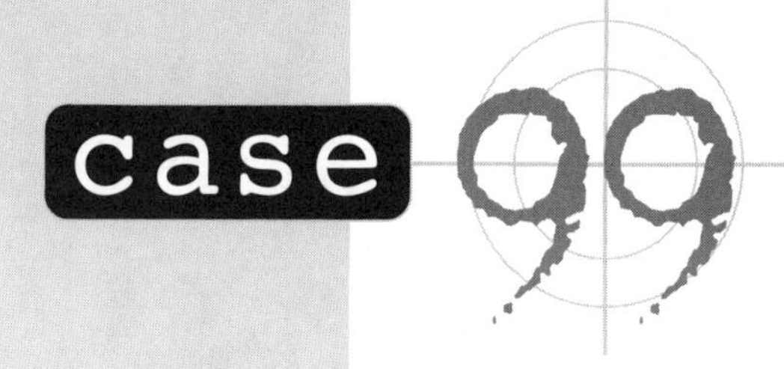

case 99

ID/CC A 3-year-old girl is brought into the genetics department for a karyotype study.

HPI She was born of a **45-year-old mother** who feels that her child is **developmentally retarded** with **characteristic "mongoloid" facial features;** her pregnancy was uneventful.

PE Generalized **hypotonia;** flattened face and low-set ears; **macroglossia;** flattened nasal bridge and **epicanthal folds;** silver-white spots on the periphery of irises (BRUSHFIELD SPOTS); single **transverse palmar crease** (SIMIAN CREASE); widely split fixed S2 (due to an atrial septic defect).

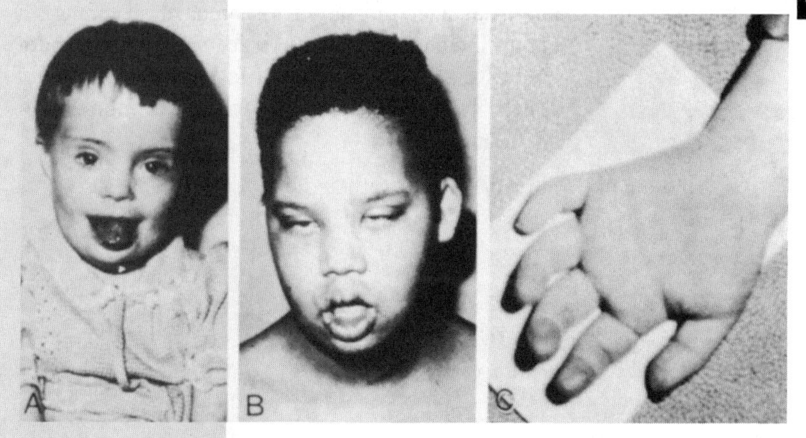

Figure 99-1. Flat broad face; oblique palpebral fissures: epicanthus: and furrowed lower lip.

Labs Karyotype: **47,XX; trisomy 21.**

Imaging KUB: **double bubble** (dilated stomach and proximal duodenum) due to **duodenal atresia.** XR, plain: hypoplastic middle and terminal phalanges of fifth digits (ACROMICRIA). Echo: endocardial cushion defect.

Gross Pathology Brachycephalic head; small brain with shallow sulci; hypoplasia of frontal sinuses; endocardial cushion defect.

case 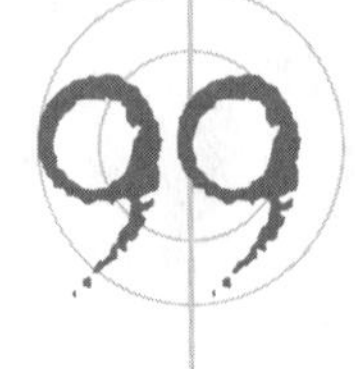

Down Syndrome

Differential

Fragile X syndrome
Trisomy 18
Fetal alcohol syndrome
Carbohydrate metabolism defects
Zellweger syndrome
Lysosomal storage disease

Discussion

The **most common chromosomal disorder,** Down syndrome is most frequently caused by trisomy 21 (due to nondisjunction); it is less commonly caused by mosaicism or a Robertsonian translocation. It is associated with a higher incidence with **advanced maternal age** (indication for prenatal screening); a higher incidence of cardiac defects, especially **endocardial cushion defects;** and a higher incidence of **acute leukemia** and **presenile dementia of Alzheimer type.**

Treatment

Surgery for congenital heart defects and duodenal atresia; training in specialized groups.

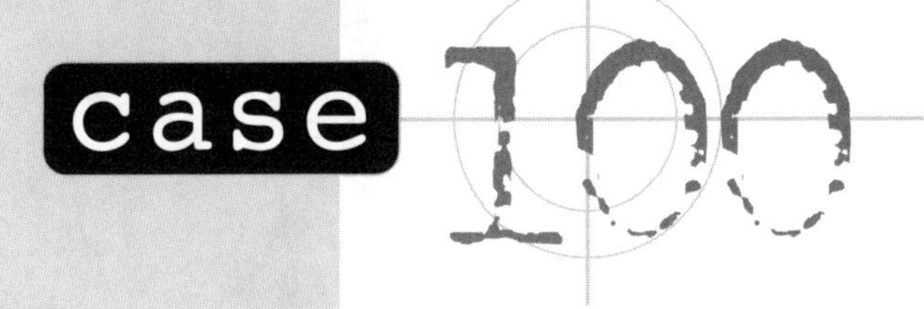

case 100

ID/CC A 7-year-old boy is brought to the optometrist for **diminished visual acuity** and requests a prescription for eyeglasses.

HPI The boy has an unusual body habitus with long arms and legs; a family history reveals similar body proportions in other family members.

PE Tall; **long extremities;** arm span greater than height (DOLICHOSTENOMELIA); **long, slender fingers** (ARACHNODACTYLY); **dislocation of lenses** (ECTOPIA LENTIS); severe myopia; inguinal hernia; high-arched palate; flat feet (PES PLANUS); **aortic diastolic murmur** (aortic insufficiency).

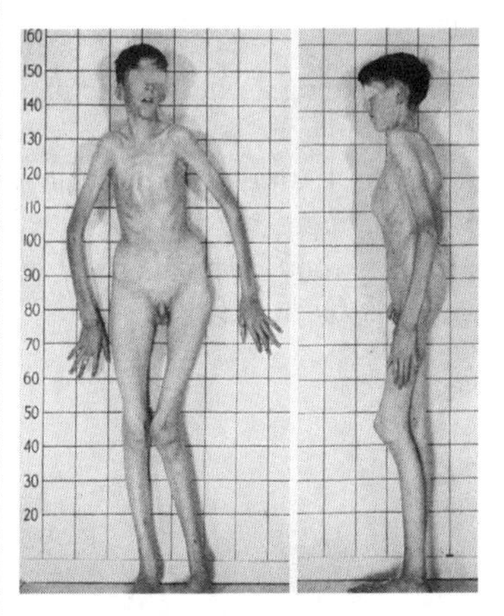

Figure 100-1. Arachnodactyly, relatively long limbs (dolichostenomelia), pectus carinatum, and pes planus.

Labs Fibrillin gene mutation identified on molecular studies.

Imaging CXR/CT/MR: marked dilatation of ascending aorta. XR, plain: thoracic and lumbar kyphoscoliosis. Echo: **mitral valve prolapse.**

Micro Pathology **Cystic medial necrosis** of aorta may lead to **dissection, rupture, aneurysm**, or **aortic insufficiency.**

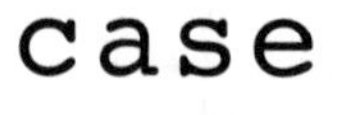
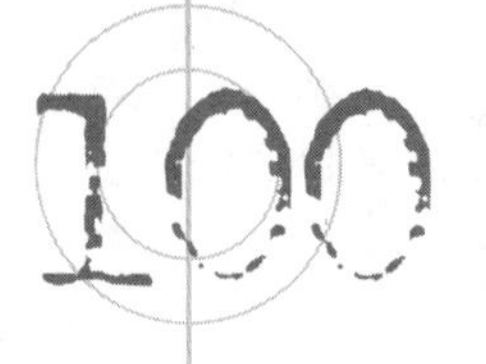

Marfan Syndrome

Differential

Ehlers–Danlos syndrome
Gigantism
Klinefelter syndrome
XXY syndrome
Long-chain acyl-CoA dehydrogenase deficiency
Sleep apnea

Discussion

A systemic connective tissue disease characterized by an **autosomaldominant** pattern of inheritance, Marfan syndrome is due to a defective chromosome 15 **fibrillin gene,** a glycoprotein secreted by fibroblasts that acts as a scaffolding for the deposition of elastin.

Treatment

Spine bracing; ophthalmologic correction; endocarditis prophylaxis; beta-blockers to slow enlargement of aortic root; annual echocardiograms to evaluate aortic root diameter; composite valve graft replacement of aortic root when diameter exceeds 55 mm; aortic valve replacement.

questions

1. A 52-year-old woman visits her family physician with complaints of progressive dyspnea on exertion, and easy fatigue. She often feels "faint" after walking long distances. Her family physician appreciates a crescendo-decrescendo systolic ejection murmur at the second intercoastal space. Which of the following most likely contributes to the development of this condition?

   A. Tertiary syphilis
   B. Atherosclerosis
   C. Congenital bicuspid valve
   D. Hyperthyroidism
   E. Coxsackie B infection

2. A 56-year-old man with diabetes with a past medical history significant for hypertension, high cholesterol, and diabetes is seen in the emergency room with sharp, ripping chest pain radiating to his back. His blood pressure is found to be 80/40 and he appears faint. An ECG demonstrates no irregularities. Which other finding may be found in this patient?

   A. Total occlusion of the left main artery by coronary coarctation
   B. Elevated jugular venous pressure
   C. Elevated cardiac troponins
   D. A loud friction rub appreciated on cardiac auscultation
   E. Mediastinal widening seen on CXR

3. A 72–year-old man with a history of two myocardial infarctions is admitted to the hospital with progressive shortness of breath and swelling in his lower extremities. He also describes having difficulty sleeping on his back without feeling short of breath. A CXR demonstrates an enlarged cardiac shadow and bilateral pleural effusions. Which of the following exam findings would most likely be seen in this patient?

   A. A third heart sound (S3)
   B. A harsh machinery murmur
   C. Carotid and femoral bruits
   D. A low-pitched mid-diastolic murmur
   E. A low-pitched "plop" during early diastole

4. A 19-year-old man, who is otherwise healthy, presents to the emergency room. He is brought by ambulance after collapsing on the field during football practice. His coach notes that the patient complained of shortness of breath and chest pain prior to collapsing. The patient's brother died several years ago during a high school basketball game. Which of the following is a likely characteristic pathologic finding in this patient?

   A. Foam cells within vessel walls
   B. Stellate mesenchymal cells in an acid mucopolysacchride matrix
   C. "Onion skinning" of vessel walls
   D. The presence of heart failure cells within the alveoli of the lung
   E. Myocytes that have actin fibers in disarray

5. A 53-year-old man with pancreatic cancer undergoes an echocardiogram prior to consideration for surgery for the removal of his early-stage cancer. The study demonstrates small friable vegetations on the valve leaflets. As well, as part of his pre-surgical workup, he is found to have an elevated prothrombin and partial thromboplastin time. Which of the following likely accounts for the vascular findings?

   A. Aortic stenosis
   B. Libman–Sacks endocarditis
   C. Bacterial endocarditis
   D. Murantic endocarditis
   E. Rheumatic heart disease

6. An unidentified homeless man is transferred to a Midwest county hospital after being found slumped on a bus stop on one of the coldest nights of the year. The patient is unarousable with a "thready" pulse. A rectal temperature demonstrates a core temperature of 27.8°C. Which of the following may also be appreciated in this patient?

   A. Bilateral papilledema
   B. Sinus tachycardia
   C. Low-voltage QRS complex on ECG
   D. Osborn waves on ECG
   E. No discernable p waves seen on ECG

7. A 67-year-old retired farmer is seen by his family physician for a physical examination. The patient notes no significant changes in his health other than the development of a slow-growing lesion on his right cheek. After a thorough examination the physician suspects a basal cell carcinoma and refers the patient to a dermatologist. Which of the following is true regarding this lesion?

A. Results from a type IV hypersensitivity reaction
B. Can often develop into malignant melanoma
C. Often associated with gluten sensitivity and enteropathy
D. May progress to squamous cell carcinoma
E. Usually appears as a pearly papule with superficial telangectasias

8. A 3–year-old child is brought to the emergency room with an erythematous rash prominent on the palms and soles. On exam, the child has significant conjunctival injection and palpably enlarged cervical lymph nodes along with a fever of 102°F. After ruling out numerous other causes, a working diagnosis of Kawasaki disease is made. This disease of vascular origin can present with which of the following?

A. Aneurysms of coronary arteries
B. Occluded segments of small and medium vessels of the arms and legs
C. Aneurismal dilation of the aortic root
D. "Onion skinning" of the renal arterioles
E. Cordlike inflammation at the site of intravenous infusion

9. A 15-year-old girl is brought to the dermatologist for a week-long rash. She notes the rash is scaly, red, mildly pruritic, raised and primarily on the neck, trunk and upper extremities. She notes that the rash started with a small oval lesion on her upper arm, but has spread since then. She denies any other medical conditions, taking any new medications, new detergent use, or consuming any new or unusual foods. Given the history, the rash is most likely that of?

A. Psoriasis
B. Syphilis
C. Pyoderma gangrenosum
D. Pityriasis rosea
E. Stevens–Johnson syndrome

10. An otherwise healthy African American man presents to his family physician for a routine physical exam. The patient complains of an enlarging area of "white pigmentation" developing on his left knee and right elbow. He denies the use of any new medications or the application of any topical preparations to the area. What would a biopsy of the affected area likely demonstrate?

A. Monro microabscesses
B. Wickham striae
C. Pautrier abscesses
D. Loss of cohesion of epidermal cells
E. Absence of melanocytes

11. A 66-year-old man notes occasional blood in his urine. He denies any pain or difficulty with urination. He is a heavy smoker with an approximate 75 pack-year history of tobacco use. His genital exam shows normal descended testicles bilaterally and a circumcised phallus. His digital rectal exam displays a mildly enlarged prostate without nodules. He has no palpable bony tenderness along his spine. His symptoms are most concerning for which of the following?

A. Nephrolithiasis
B. Bladder cancer
C. Benign prostatic hypertrophy
D. Prostate cancer
E. IgA nephropathy

12. A 16-year-old boy is seen in the emergency room after his mother learns that he has been coughing up blood for a couple of days. As well, the boy notes that he has also been urinating dark orange. The emergency room physician suspects Goodpasture syndrome and immediately starts intravenous steroids and admits the patient for a kidney biopsy. What would be the likely finding of such a biopsy?

A. Increased mesangeal matrix deposition with nodules formation in the mesangium
B. "Wire loops" as a result of subendothelial immunocomplex deposition
C. "Lumpy bumpy" immunofluorescense seen in the glomeruli
D. Linear IgG deposition along the glomerular basement membrane by immunofluorescence
E. Apple green birefringence of the mesangium when viewed with polarized light

13. A 24-year-old man presents to his family physician with complaints of a "swollen testicle." He notes that it has been enlarging for the past few months. He specifically denies any recent sexual encounters. On physical examination, a firm mass is palpated in the left hemiscrotum. The mass is nontender and does not transilluminate. A battery of serum markers, including α-fetoprotein, LDH, and B-HcG are all within the normal limits. The patient is referred to an urologist who performs an orchiectomy. The pathology will likely reveal?

A. Choriocarcinoma
B. Mixed germ cell neoplasm
C. Testicular torsion
D. Dysgerminoma
E. Semioma

14. A 2-year-old girl is brought to the pediatrician by her mother as she is concerned that the infant has developed an "enlarging belly." The physician is able to detect a large abdominal mass on physical examination. Labs demonstrate a normal vanyllylmandelic acid level, and a referral is made to a pediatric surgeon to obtain a biopsy. A diagnosis is made and the patient is found to have Wilms tumor. Which of the following was found on laboratory analysis or pathologic biopsy?

A. Multiple fluid-filled cysts in the kidney
B. Presence of blastemic, stromal, and epithelial cell types
C. Horner–Wright pseudorosettes
D. Flexner–Wintersteiner rosettes
E. Cryptorchidism

15. A 9-year-old boy visits his family physician with his mother. He complains of sudden onset of pain in his left hip. The mother also notes that he has developed a limp. The boy is well above the 95th percentile for weight and only 15th percentile for height. He denies any trauma to the leg. X-rays are ordered demonstrating that the left leg is extremely rotated and 2 cm shorter than the controlateral leg. Given the clinical and radiographic findings, the boy is thought to have a slipped femoral epiphyses. Which of the following might be the long-term sequelae of such a condition?

A. Anterior cruciate ligament injury
B. Femoral fracture
C. Osteoarthritis
D. Dupuytren contracture
E. Septic arthritis

16. An 18-year-old boy is referred to an orthopaedic surgeon for concern of progressive swelling above the right knee. The patient denies any previous trauma to the region. X-ray of the involved region demonstrates a periosteal elevation, which on the radiographic report is described as Codman triangle. A likely diagnosis of osteosarcoma is made and the patient is scheduled for surgery. Which of the following would not be surprising if they were a part of the patient's medical history?

A. Retinoblastoma
B. Paget disease of the bone
C. Ewing sarcoma
D. Sickle cell anemia
E. Barrett esophagus

17. A 2-year-old child is brought to the emergency room because of complaints of a "really bad belly ache." The mother tells the emergency room physician that the child has been passing "red currant jelly" stools. On exam, an oblong abdominal mass is palpated. A barium enema shows telescoping of the ileum into the cecum. After the diagnostic test the patient no longer complains of abdominal pain. What was the likely condition?

A. Pyloric stenosis
B. Appendicitis
C. Meckel diverticulum
D. Abdominal aortic aneurysm
E. Intussusception

18. A 16-year-old boy presents with severe right lower quadrant abdominal pain, anorexia, nausea, vomiting, and low-grade fever. The pain started 24 hours ago in the periumbilical region, but has now migrated to McBurney point. He has not sustained any trauma to the area. The patient is lying very still on the bed. On abdominal examination, the obdurate sign is elicited, and rebound tenderness and involuntary guarding are present in the right lower quadrant of the abdomen. The patient is sent to the operating room for an appendectomy. If the surgical specimen were to be sent for pathologic analysis, which of the following would most likely be seen?

A. Granulation tissue, with areas of fibrosis and new vessel formation
B. An abscess, with neutrophilic infiltration
C. Liquifarctive necrosis
D. Multinucleated Langerhans giant cells and central caseous necrosis
E. Massivē infiltration of lymphocytes with germinal center formation

19. A young girl presents to the physician's office for a sports physical before participation in volleyball. She appears to have a perfect habitus for the sport as she is much taller than her peers and has exceptionally long arms and fingers. Upon auscultation of her heart there is a midsystolic click associated with a murmur of mitral valve prolapse. The physician suspects she may have Marfan syndrome, a defect in which of the following proteins?

A. Myosin heavy chain
B. Spectrin or ankrin
C. Dystrophin
D. Fibrillen
E. Collagen

20. A 17-year-old boy who displays the typical features of Down syndrome, including prominent epicanthal folds, brushfield spots, a large protruding tongue, and a simian crease, is seen by his primary care physician. Although he is healthy, his family has been reading and is concerned about the possibility to develop which of the following conditions?

A. Lymphoblastic leukemia
B. Berry aneurysm of the circle of Willis
C. Osteosarcoma involving the proximal tibia
D. A "pill-rolling" tremor
E. Carcinoma of the thyroid

answers

1-C

A. Tertiary syphilis [Incorrect] This is associated with several pathologic findings of which aortitis is one. However, involvement of the aortic valve leads to insufficiency with a diastolic decrescendo murmur.

B. Atherosclerosis [Incorrect] This is a major contributor to coronary artery disease, which can lead to myocardial infarction.

C. Congenital bicuspid valve [Correct] Calcification of the aortic valve occurs earlier in life in patients with a congenital bicuspid valve leading to aortic stenosis with the characteristically described murmur.

D. Hyperthyroidism [Incorrect] Although hyperthyroidism may be associated with the development of atrial fibrillation with an appreciable irregularly irregular heart beat, it is not associated with valvular heart disease.

E. Coxsackie virus B [Incorrect] This virus is associated with myocarditis, which is rarely audibly appreciated; rather it can cause ECG changes.

2-E

A. Total occlusion of the left main artery [Incorrect]. This would result in a significant myocardial infarction that would be evident on an ECG as ST elevations.

B. Elevated jugular venous pressure [Incorrect] Patients who are volume overloaded, as in congestive heart failure, have an elevated jugular venous pressure. Just the opposite, volume depletion, is evident in significant hypotension.

C. Elevated cardiac troponins [Incorrect] Damage to cardiac cells results in the elevation of enzymes such as cardiac troponins as may happen in myocardial infarction or myocarditis.

D. A loud friction rub appreciated on cardiac auscultation [Incorrect] This can be associated with pericarditis.

E. Mediatinal widening seen on CXR [Correct] The patient in the case has an aortic dissection, with the leakage of blood from the aorta into the mediastinum. A CXR would demonstrate widening of the mediastinum.

3-A

A. A third heart sound (S3) [Correct] This is the sound of the atrium contracting to help pump blood in the weakened heart (atrial kick) of the patient with congestive heart failure (as in this patient).

B. A harsh machinery murmur [Incorrect] Failure of the ductus arteriosum to close during birth results in a persistent ductus arteriosum. On exam, these patients have a harsh machinery murmur.

C. Carotid and femoral bruits [Incorrect] These can be appreciated in patients with significant atherosclerotic disease. Turbid blood flow through the large vessels creates a low pitched rumbling (bruit).

D. A low pitched mid-diastolic murmur [Incorrect] This is associated with mitral stenosis. The most common cause of mitral stenosis is rheumatic heart disease.

E. A low pitched "plop" during diastole [Incorrect] This results from a cardiac myxoma, the most common primary tumor of the heart. The plop is due to the tumor that acts as a ball-valve obstruction.

4-E

A. Foam cells [Incorrect] These are lipid-laden cells that are a component of the fibrous plaque that forms in vessels affected by atherosclerosis.

B. Stellate mesenchymal cells in an acid mucopolysacchride matrix [Incorrect] The most common tumors of the heart, myxomas, are composed of stellate mesenchymal cells that produce acid mucopolyssachrides.

C. "Onion skinning" of vessel walls [Incorrect] Patients with malignant hypertension have hyperplastic atherosclerosis, which histologically appears as onion skinning arterioles.

D. Heart failure cells [Incorrect] These are hemosiderin-laden macrophages that accumulate as a result of passive congestion in the lungs of patients with congestive heart failure.

E. Myocytes that have actin fibers in disarray [Correct] Patients with idiopathic hypertrophic subaortic stenosis have an autosomal dominant defect in the B-myosin heavy chain resulting in a histologically characteristic disarray of actin fibers in myocytes.

5-D

A. Aortic stenosis [Incorrect] This is associated with calcium deposition within the aortic valve and is often associated with a congenital bicuspid valve.
B. Libman–Sacks endocarditis [Incorrect] This is a complication of systemic lupus erythematosis (SLE) in which verrucous vegetations develop on the underside of the mitral valve.
C. Bacterial endocarditis [Incorrect] This results in larger, friable, nonsterile vegetations and is often due to *Staphyloccocus aureus* or *Streptococcus viridans*.
D. Murantic endocarditis [Correct] Also known as nonbacterial thrombotic endocarditis (NBTE), this occurs in patients with cancers as pancreatic cancer. These people are hypercoagulable and form small sterile thrombi on the valves.
E. Rheumatic heart disease [Incorrect] This is the leading cause of mitral stenosis, which is not associated with vegetations on the heart valves.

6-D

A. Bilateral papilledema [Incorrect] Patients with malignant hypertension have severely elevated blood pressures leading to end organ damage of the brain and kidneys. Patients may present with bilateral papilledema.
B. Sinus tachycardia [Incorrect] This is a rather nonspecific finding that occurs in several conditions, including physiologic exercise, dehydration, arrhythmia, etc. However, a hypothermic patient would likely be bradycardiac.
C. Low-voltage QRS complexes on ECG [Incorrect] Patients who have constrictive pericarditis due to tuberculosis, radiation exposure, rheumatic conditions, or uremia have low-voltage QRS complexes on ECG.
D. Osborn waves [Correct] Also known as J waves, Osborn waves are upward waves immediately following the S wave on an ECG. Although not completely specific in patients in hypothermia, they can be found in this patient.
E. No discernable p waves present on an ECG [Incorrect] Patients with rapid atrial fibrillation, who are not rate controlled, have no discernable p waves present on an ECG.

7-E

A. Type IV hypersensitivity reaction [Incorrect] Contact dermatitis usually presents as pruritic vesicles that weep and encrust. The mechanism of contact dermatitis is clearly a type IV cell-mediated hypersensitivity reaction.

B. Malignant melanoma [Incorrect] Basal cell carcinomas are rarely if ever malignant; however, patients with dysplastic nevus syndrome often have numerous dysplastic nevi that can develop into malignant melanoma.

C. Gluten sensitivity enteropathy [Incorrect] Patients with this condition often have a pruritic rash on the knees, elbows, and back with subepidermal blisters. This disorder, dermatitis herpatiformis, results from IgA deposition at the tips of dermal papillae and localized immune reactions.

D. Squamous cell carcinoma [Incorrect] Actinic keratosis presents as tan plaques on areas of prolonged sun exposure. These lesions must be biopsied as they can progress to squamous cell carcinoma.

E. Pearly papule with superficial telangectasias [Correct] Basal cell carcinoma usually presents as pearly papules with superficial telangectasias or pearly papules with rolled borders and central ulcerations.

8-A

A. Aneurysms of coronary arteries [Correct] Kawasaki disease is an arteritis involving large, medium-sized, and small arteries (often the coronary arteries). A feared complication of this disorder is an aneurysm of the coronary arteries, which can rupture or thrombose leading to a myocardial infarction with sudden death.

B. Occluded segments of small and medium vessels of the arms and legs [Incorrect] Thromboangitis obliterans is an arteritis of medium-sized and small arteries of the tibial and radial arteries of the arms and legs. It can result in claudication of the legs and gangrene distal extremities.

C. Aneurismal dilation of the aortic root [Incorrect] A complication of tertiary syphilis is the aneurismal dilation of the aortic root. This can result in severe aortic valve incompetence.

D. "Onion skinning" of the renal arterioles [Incorrect] Patients with malignant hypertension develop hyperplastic atherosclerosis that appears as "onion skinning" of the renal arterioles. This ultimately results in luminal obliveration with ischemic changes in the involved glomeruli.

E. Cordlike inflammation at the site of intravenous infusion [Incorrect] Patients who have indwelling venous catheters develop superficial thrombophlebitis, characterized by cordlike inflammation of the site of intravenous infusion.

9-D

A. Psoriasis [Incorrect] This usually presents as salmon-colored plaques with overlying silver scales. The condition is typically hereditary and confined to the extremities, particularly extensor surfaces.
B. Syphilis [Incorrect] Syphilis is a sexually transmitted disease that initially presents as a chancre and then recedes only to present weeks later with a macule-papule rash on the palms and soles.
C. Pyoderma gangrenosum [Incorrect] Patients with inflammatory bowel disease or leukemia, may present with an ulcerlike lesion on the extremities. This condition, pyoderma gangreosum, is treated with systemic steroids.
D. Pityriasis rosea [Correct] This patient presents with a classic case of pityriasis rosea. This rash is common in teenagers and often presents with a single lesion (herald patch) followed by extension to involve the trunk, neck, and upper extremities.
E. Stevens–Johnson syndrome [Incorrect] This is an erosive crusting of the lips and oral mucosa that results as an idiosyncratic reaction to medications.

10-E

A. Monro microabscesses [Incorrect] Biopsies from patients with psoriasis would demonstrate collections of polymorphonuclear cells (PMNs) within the stratum corneum (Monro abscesses).
B. Wickham striae [Incorrect] These are visible tiny white dots and lines over the papules of the lesions in patients with lichen planus.
C. Pautrier abscesses [Incorrect] Mycosis fungoides, a malignant cutaneous helper T-cell lymphoma, is characterized by a skin biopsy that microscopically reveals dermal infiltrates with atypical mononuclear cells appearing as epidermal microabscesses, known as Pautrier abscess.
D. Loss of cohesion of epidermal cells [Incorrect] Pemphigus vulgaris is a serious intraepidermal blistering disorder characterized by the loss of cohesion of epidermal cells, known as acatholysis.

E. Absence of melanocytes [Correct] Vitiligo, as in the case of this presentation, is believed to be an autoimmune disorder characterized by destruction of melanocytes. The destruction leads to the absence of pigmentation in the involved region due to the lack of melanocytes.

11-B

A. Nephrolithiasis [Incorrect] This often presents with flank pain radiating to the groin. As well, patients often present with hemoturia due to trauma to the ureter as the stone passes.
B. Bladder cancer [Correct] The presence of hematuria, both microscopic and gross, in men is concerning for bladder cancer. This patient has an impressive tobacco history, a known risk factor for the development of bladder cancer.
C. Benign prostatic hypertrophy (BPH) [Incorrect] BPH typically presents with urinary symptoms of nocturia and difficulty urinating. Although the patient may indeed have findings consistent with BPH, he is asymptomatic.
D. Prostate cancer [Incorrect] The patient does not have any palpable nodularity to his prostate, to indicate prostate cancer. However, a prostate-specific antigen level would be indicated. Hematuria is not a common finding with prostate cancer. However, involvement of the seminal vesicles can result in hematuria.
E. IgA nephropathy [Incorrect] This can indeed cause hematuria. It is a renal manifestation of Berger disease. Patients often have bouts of hematuria associated with an upper respiratory infection.

12-D

A. Increased mesangeal matrix deposition with nodules formation in the mesangium [Incorrect] Patients with long-standing, poorly controlled diabetes often develop diabetic nephropathy. This condition is characterized histologically by the formation of the Kimmelsteil–Wilson nodules, composed of mesangial matrix.
B. "Wire loops" [Incorrect] Patients with involvement of the kidney in systemic lupus erythematous develop characteristic glomerular lesions. These lesions result from subendothelial immune complex depositions forming what are known as "wire loops."

C. "Lumpy bumpy" immunofluorescense seen in the glomeruli [Incorrect] The most common form of the nephrotic syndrome is membraneous glomerulonephritis. In this disease entity a biopsy of the kidney would demonstrate "lumpy bumpy" immunofluorescence as a result of the nonspecific deposition of immune complexes in the glomeruli.

D. Linear IgG deposition along the glomerular basement membrane by immunofluorescence [Correct] Patients with Goodpasture syndrome develop autoantibodies to specific antigens on glomerular and basement membranes. This results in Type II hypersensitivity with localized damage to the tissues. A biopsy would reveal linear IgG deposition along such membranes.

E. Apple green birefringence of the mesangium when viewed with polarized light [Incorrect] Patients with amyloidosis deposit amyloid protein in numerous organs including the kidney. This amyloid is detected by staining with Congo Red stains. The presence of amyloid is detected by apple green birefringence visualized on polarized microscopy.

13-C

A. Choriocarcinomas [Incorrect] These are highly malignant testicular neoplasms. They often only present as small, barely palpable masses, before widely metastasizing. As they are composed of cytotrophoblasts and synciotrophoblasts, they produce detectable levels of B-HcG.

B. Mixed germ cell neoplasm [Incorrect] The majority of testicular tumors are not "pure" tumors, but rather mixed germ cell neoplasms. Typically, these tumors produce products of the elements of mixed into the tumor, including B-HcG (choriocarcinoma) and α-fetoprotein (endodermal sinus tumors).

C. Testicular torsion [Incorrect] This is often an acute painful condition that occurs as a result of twisting of the spermatic cord. The arteries usually remain patent, but the veins become compressed resulting in vessel engorgement of the testicles.

D. Dysgerminomas [Incorrect] These are the histologic equivalent to the seminomas in female patients. They are relatively uncommon in females and, like seminomas, are extremely radiosensitive.

E. Seminomas [Correct] These are the most common type of germ cell tumor in males. They do not produce products like B-HcG or α-fetoprotein. They often present as painless swelling of the testicles. They are treated with surgery followed by radiation to at-risk lymph nodes.

14-B

A. Multiple fluid-filled cysts in the kidney [Incorrect] Adult polycystic kidney disease is an autosomal dominant disorder characterized by dramatically enlarged kidneys appreciated as a nontender mass in adults. The kidney is filled with multiple fluid-filled cysts.

B. Presence of blastemic, stromal, and epithelial cell types [Correct] Wilms tumor is the most common tumor of the kidney in children. This small round blue cell tumor demonstrates the presence of cells attempting to recapitulate different stages of nephrogenesis including blastemic, stromal, and epithelial types.

C. Horner–Wright pseudorosettes [Incorrect] Yet another potential cause of an enlarging abdominal mass in a young child is a neuroblastoma. This tumor of the adrenal results in the overproduction of catelcholamines, evidenced by increased urinary vanillylmandelic acid (VMA). This tumor is characterized by the presence of distinct Horner–Wright pseudorosettes.

D. Flexner–Wintersteiner rosettes [Incorrect] Retinoblastoma is another "small round blue cell tumor" as is neuroblastoma and Wilms tumor. This tumor of the retina has the distinctive microscopic appearance including the presence of Flexner–Wintersteiner rosettes.

E. Cryptorchidism [Incorrect] This is the failure of the testis to descend into the scrotum during development. Cryptorchidism even when surgically corrected confers an added risk of the development of germ cell neoplasm in males.

15-C

A. Anterior cruciate ligament injury [Incorrect] Athletes are at most risk of developing anterior cruciate ligament injury, which occurs as in the case of a fall on a hyperextended knee and can often be appreciated by a "popping" noise in the knee during the injury. Patients have a positive anterior drawer sign appreciated on physical exam

B. Femoral fracture [Incorrect] This is often associated with osteoporosis in older women. Additional risk factors include avascular necrosis of the hip, steroid therapy, sickle cell anemia, and radiation therapy.

C. Osteoarthritis [Correct] Slipped femoral epiphyses is most common in overweight males. The treatment includes surgical fixation. Patients are at increased risk for the development of avascular necrosis of the femoral head and early osteoarthritis.

D. Duputyren contracture [Incorrect] This is associated with alcoholism and manual labor. It results in an inability to extend the fourth and fifth fingers.
E. Septic arthritis [Incorrect] Septic arthritis in children is most often due to hematogenous spread rather than compromise of the joint due to injury. The most common cause of septic arthritis in children is *Staphyloccocus aureus.*

16-A

A. Retinoblastoma [Correct] Patients with hereditary mutations in the retinoblastoma gene have hundreds-fold risk for the development of osteosarcoma. Therefore, it is not unlikely to hear that the patient had an eye enucleated because of retinoblastoma.
B. Paget disease of bone [Incorrect] This is indeed associated with the development of osteosarcoma, however, less so than retinoblastoma. As well, Paget disease of the bone is a disease of older men that is characterized by bone pain and bone overgrowth.
C. Ewing sarcoma [Incorrect] This is another type of bone tumor that is a type of small round blue cell tumor. It is associated with the translocation t(11;22). It often arises in the femur and flat bones of the pelvis.
D. Sickle cell anemia [Incorrect] Patients with sickle cell anemia are at increased risk of avascular necrosis of bone. As well, they have an increased incidence of osteomyelitis as opposed to the general population.
E. Barrett esophagus [Incorrect] A common predisposing factor in the development of esophageal carcinoma is the development of Barrett esophagus. It, however, has no relation to bone tumors.

17-E

A. Pyloric stenosis [Incorrect] Patients with pyloric stenosis usually present early after birth with nonbillous vomiting. An ovoid mass can be palpated in the abdomen. Surgical correction is required to remove hypertrophic tissue from around the pylorus.
B. Appendicitis [Incorrect] Surgical resection is required as well for appendicitis. There is no abdominal mass appreciated, and there is palpable reproducible RLQ pain. Enemas are contraindicated because of the risk of perforation.
C. Meckel diverticulum [Incorrect] This is a common finding in approximately 2% of the population. It is a small patch in the intestine and usually asymptomatic, although bleeding and ulceration may occur. Such diverticula can also be seen as lead points for the development of intussusception.

D. Abdominal aortic aneurysm [Incorrect] An abdominal aortic aneurysm can be appreciated as a pulsating painless upper abdominal mass. However, as atherosclerotic disease is usually the cause, this patient would not have this condition.
E. Intussusception [Correct] Telescoping of bowel segment inside of another occurs in intussusception. Often there is an identifiable lead part such as a hyperplastic Peyer patch or Meckel diverticulum. A barium enema is both diagnostic and therapeutic.

18-B

A. Granulation tissue [Incorrect] Such tissue is formed during wound healing and consists of newly formed capillaries and young fibroblasts.
B. An abscess with neutrophilic infiltration [Correct] This is a case of acute inflammation in appendicitis. Neutrophils are the primary effector cells present in acute inflammatory infiltrates, inducing pus formation and an abscess.
C. Liquifarctive necrosis [Incorrect] This occurs primarily in the brain. It can occur after a cerebrovascular accident or in cases of brain abscesses.
D. Multinucleated Langerhans giant cells and central caseous necrosis [Incorrect] These occur with forms of granulomatous inflammation as with tuberculosis.
E. Massive infiltration of lymphocytes with germinal center formation [Incorrect] In cases of diseases like Hashimoto thyroisitis or Sjögren syndrome, it is not uncommon to find massive infiltration of lymphocytes with germinal center formation.

19-D

A. Myosin heavy chain [Incorrect] Familial hypertroic cardiomyopathy is associated with defects in mysosin heavy chain.
B. Myosin heavy chain [Incorrect] Hereditary spherocytosis with mutations in spectrin or secondary defects in ankrin.
C. Dystrophin [Incorrect] This is a large structural protein important in muscle cells, deficiency leads to muscular dystrophy.
D. Fibrillen [Correct] Marfan disease presents similar to the case described and results from an autosomal dominant mutation in the structural protein fibrillin.
E. Collagen [Incorrect] Collagen defects are seen in Ehler–Danlos syndrome and vitamin C deficiency.

20-A

A. Lymphoblastic leukemia [Correct] Patients with Down syndrome are at increased susceptibility to developing lymphoblastic leukemia, as well as Alzheimer disease.

B. Berry aneurysm of the circle of Willis [Incorrect]. This is common in patients with polycyctic kidney disease.

C. Osteosarcoma involving the proximal tibia [Incorrect] Osteosarcoma is more common in patients with a history of retinoblastoma as well as in patients with a history of Paget disease of bone.

D. A "pill-rolling tremor" [Incorrect] This is the description for patients with Parkinson disease, which unlike Alzheimer disease is not associated with Down syndrome.

E. Carcinoma of the thyroid [Incorrect] This is associated with exposure to radiation or with multiple endocrine neoplasia syndromes or mutations in the RET oncogene.

credits

Anatomical Chart Company (asset for Case 82).

Austen KF, Frank MM, et al. *Samter's Immunologic Diseases*. 6th Ed. Philadelphia: Lippincott Williams & Wilkins, 2001. Fig. 44.4 (Case 22).

Becker KL, Bilezikian JP, Brenner WJ, et al. *Principles and Practice of Endocrinology and Metabolism*. 3rd Ed. Philadelphia: Lippincott Williams & Wilkins, 2001. Figs. 150-1B (Case 58), 111-9 (Case 71), 215-20 (Case 60).

Berg D, Worzala K. *Atlas of Adult Physical Diagnosis*. Philadelphia: Lippincott Williams & Wilkins, 2005. Fig. 8.23 (Case 81).

Bhushan V, Le T, Pall V. *Underground Clinical Vignettes: Step One—Pathophysiology III*. 4th Ed. Malden, Mass: Blackwell Publishing, 2005. Figs. 003 (Case 3), 035 (Case 35), 036 (Case 36), 043 (Case 43), 051 (Case 51), 065 (Case 65), 070 (Case 70).

Bickley LS, Szilagyi P. *Bates' Guide to Physical Examination and History Taking*. 8th Ed. Philadelphia: Lippincott Williams & Wilkins, 2003. (Case 82).

Chapman MW. *Chapman's Orthopaedic Surgery*. 3rd Ed. Philadelphia: Lippincott Williams & Wilkins. Figs. 62.2 (Case 78), 154.8.A (Case 86).

DeVita VT, Hellman S, Rosenberg SA. *Cancer: Principles and Practice of Oncology*. Philadelphia: Lippincott Williams & Wilkins, 2004. Figs. 37-10B (Case 32), 24.1.1 (Case 66).

Eisenberg RL. *Clinical Imaging: An Atlas of Differential Diagnosis*. 4th Ed. Philadelphia: Lippincott Williams & Wilkins. Figs. GU 16-4 (Case 57), GU 32-12 (Case 68), CA 18-2 (Case 69), B 4-13 (Case 77), B 24-1 (Case 79), GI 74-2B (Case 96).

Fishman MC, Hoffman AR, et al. *Medicine*. 5th Ed. Philadelphia: Lippincott Williams & Wilkins, 2003. Fig. 4-2 (Case 2).

Gillenwater JY, Grayhack JT, et al. *Adult and Pediatric Urology*. 4th Ed. Philadelphia: Lippincott Williams & Wilkins, 2001. Figs. 20.2 (Case 52), 3E.23 (Case 56), 16.2 (Case 67), 53.13 (Case 74).

Goodheart HP. *Goodheart's Photoguide of Common Skin Disorders.* 2nd Ed. Philadelphia: Lippincott Williams & Wilkins, 2003. Fig. 2.11 (Case 31).

Goroll AH, Mulley AG. *Primary Care Medicine: Office Evaluation and Management of the Adult Patient.* 5th Ed. Philadelphia: Lippincott, Williams & Wilkins, 2005. Figs. 177-4 (Case 30), 177-8 (Case 41).

Grammer LC, Greenberger PA. *Patterson's Allergic Diseases.* 6th Ed. Philadelphia: Lippincott Williams & Wilkins, 2002. Fig. 18.1 (Case 33).

Green GB, Harris IS, et al. The *Washington Manual of Medical Therapeutics,* 31st ed. Philadelphia: Lippincott Williams & Wilkins, 2004. T9-2. Fig. 10-1 (Case 10).

Greenberg MJ, Hendrickson RG. *Greenberg's Text-Atlas of Emergency Medicine.* Philadelphia: Lippincott, Williams & Wilkins, 2004. Figs. 7-6A & B (Case 10), 7-39 (Case 25), 16-12 (Case 39), 7-10A (Case 87), 9-36C (Case 88), 16-38B (Case 95).

Hall JC. *Sauer's Manual of Skin Disorders.* 9th Ed. Philadelphia: Lippincott Williams & Wilkins, 2006. Fig. 21-4 (Case 37).

Humes HD. *Kelley's Textbook of Internal Medicine.* 2nd Ed. Philadelphia: Lippincott Williams & Wilkins, 2001. Figs. 78.9 (Case 14), 150.2A (Case 59), 150.10.B (Case 62), 150.8 (Case 63), 150.7D (Case 64), 412.2C (Case 84).

Irwin RS, Rippe JM. *Irwin & Rippe's Intensive Care Medicine.* 5th Ed. Philadelphia: Lippincott Williams & Wilkins. Figs. 65-1 (Case 17), 42-11 (Case 29).

Kelsen DP, Daly JM, Kern SE, et al. *Gastrointestinal Oncology: Principles and Practice.* Philadelphia: Lippincott Williams & Wilkins, 2002. Fig. 24.11 (Case 92).

Koopman WJ, Moreland LW. *Arthritis and Allied Conditions: A Textbook of Rheumatology,* 15th Ed. Philadelphia: Lippincott Williams & Wilkins, 2004. Figs. 93.6 (Case 54), 96.1 (Case 100).

Lawrence PF, Bell RM, Dayton MT, et al. *Lawrence: Essentials of General Surgery.* 4th Ed. Philadelphia: Lippincott Williams & Wilkins, 2005. Fig. 23-11 (Case 23).

McMillan JA, Fergin RD, et al. *Oski's Pediatrics: Principles and Practice.* 4th Ed. Philadelphia: Lippincott Williams & Wilkins, 2006. Figs. 129.25 (Case 40), 129.56 (Case 50), 62.7 (Case 72), 313.1 (Case 73), 432.8.B (Case 80).

Mulholland MW, Lillemoe KD. *Greenfield's Surgery: Scientific Principles and Practice.* 4th Ed. Philadelphia: Lippincott Williams & Wilkins, 2005. Figs. 84.7 (Case 21), 119.18 (Case 83).

Rubin E, Farber JL. *Pathology.* 3rd Ed. Philadelphia: Lippincott Williams & Wilkins, 1999. Fig. 10-38 (Case 26).

Rubin E, Gorstein F, Schwarting R, et al. *Rubin's Pathology: A Clinicopathologic Approach.* 4th Ed. Baltimore: Lippincott Williams & Wilkins, 2004. Figs. 10-18 (Case 4), 11-48 (Case 6), 7-32 (Case 8), 11-54 (Case 9), 11-53 (Case 11), 11-29 (Case 12), 11-14 (Case 13), 11-37 (Case 19), 11-40 (Case 20), 10-36B (Case 27), 4-14 (Case 49), 16-31 (Case 53), 17-41 (Case 55), 16-47 (Case 61), 16-85 (Case 76), 18-41B (Case 93), 6-48 (Case 97).

Sadler T. *Langman's Medical Embryology.* 9th Ed. Image Bank. Baltimore: Lippincott Williams & Wilkins, 2003. Fig. 1.8A, B, C (Case 99).

Schrier RW. *Diseases of the Kidney and Urinary Tract.* 8th Ed. Philadelphia: Lippincott Williams & Wilkins, 2006. Fig. 49-3 (Case 75).

Topol EJ, Califf RM, Isner J, et al. *Textbook of Cardiovascular Medicine.* 2nd Ed. Philadelphia: Lippincott Williams & Wilkins, 2002. Figs. 47.7A (Case 1), 60.14 (Case 5), 90.4 (Case 16).

Wolfson AB, Hendey GW, et al. *Harwood-Nuss' Clinical Practice of Emergency Medicine.* 4th Ed. Philadelphia: Lippincott Williams & Wilkins, 2005. Figs. 126.11 (Case 38), 126.12 (Case 42), 126.5 (Case 44), 127.4 (Case 45), 127.2 (Case 46), 127.7 (Case 48), 68.2 (Case 89).

Yamada T, Alpers DH, et al. *Textbook of Gastroenterology.* 4th Ed. Philadelphia: Lippincott Williams & Wilkins, 2003. Figs. 49-17 (Case 34), 49-3 (Case 47), 89-7 (Case 90), 138-11 (Case 91), 152-1B (Case 94).

case list

CARDIOLOGY

1. Aortic Dissection
2. Aortic Insufficiency
3. Aortic Stenosis
4. Atherosclerosis
5. Atrial Fibrillation
6. Atrial Myxoma
7. CAD—Myocardial Infarction
8. Cardiac Tamponade
9. Cardiac Transplant
10. Congestive Heart Failure
11. Constrictive Pericarditis
12. Cor Pulmonale
13. Dilated Cardiomyopathy
14. Eisenmenger Complex
15. High-Altitude Sickness
16. Hypertrophic Cardiomyopathy
17. Hypothermia
18. Malignant Hypertension
19. Marantic Endocarditis
20. Mitral Insufficiency
21. Mitral Stenosis
22. Myocarditis
23. Peripheral Arterial Embolism
24. Shock—Hypovolemic
25. Sinus Bradycardia
26. Syphilis—Tertiary (Aortitis)
27. Thromboangiitis Obliterans—Buerger Disease
28. Thrombophlebitis—Superficial
29. Wolff–Parkinson–White Syndrome

DERMATOLOGY

30. Actinic Keratosis
31. Atopic Dermatitis
32. Basal Cell Carcinoma
33. Contact Dermatitis
34. Dermatitis Herpetiformis
35. Dysplastic Nevus Syndrome
36. Erythema Multiforme
37. Furuncle
38. Kaposi Sarcoma
39. Kawasaki Syndrome
40. Lichen Planus
41. Malignant Melanoma
42. Mycosis Fungoides
43. Osler–Weber–Rendu Syndrome
44. Pemphigus
45. Pityriasis Rosea
46. Psoriasis
47. Pyoderma Gangrenosum
48. Seborrheic Dermatitis
49. Serum Sickness
50. Vitiligo

NEPHROLOGY/UROLOGY

51. Acute Tubular Necrosis
52. Adult Polycystic Kidney Disease
53. Alport Syndrome
54. Amyloidosis—Primary
55. Benign Prostatic Hyperplasia
56. Bladder Cancer
57. Bladder Outlet Obstruction
58. Diabetic Nephropathy
59. Goodpasture Syndrome
60. Hypertensive Renal Disease
61. IgA Nephropathy
62. Lupus Nephritis
63. Membranoproliferative Glomerulonephritis

64. Membranous Glomerulonephritis
65. Minimal Change Disease
66. Prostate Carcinoma
67. Renal Cell Carcinoma
68. Renal Infarction
69. Renovascular Hypertension
70. Seminoma
71. Testicular Choriocarcinoma
72. Testicular Dysgenesis
73. Testicular Teratoma (Mixed)
74. Testicular Torsion
75. Urate Nephropathy
76. Wilms Tumor

ORTHOPEDIC

77. Ewing Sarcoma
78. Dupuytren Contracture
79. Avascular Necrosis of the Femoral Head
80. Slipped Capital Femoral Epiphysis
81. Anterior Cruciate Ligament Tear
82. Osteoarthritis
83. Osteosarcoma
84. Paget Disease of Bone
85. Septic Arthritis—Staphylococcal
86. Cervical Spondylosis

GENERAL SURGERY

87. Abdominal Aortic Aneurysm
88. Acute Cholecystitis
89. Appendicitis
90. Cecal Carcinoma
91. Esophageal Carcinoma
92. Gastric Carcinoma
93. Gastric Leiomyoma
94. Intestinal Obstruction—Acute
95. Intussusception
96. Pancreatic Carcinoma

PEDIATRICS

97. Erythroblastosis Fetalis
98. Sudden Infant Death Syndrome
99. Down Syndrome
100. Marfan Syndrome

index